Rafael Lemes de Aquino
Ailton de Souza Aragão

The impact of night work on nurses' quality of life

Rafael Lemes de Aquino
Ailton de Souza Aragão

The impact of night work on nurses' quality of life

A look at the male team

ScienciaScripts

Imprint

Cover image: www.ingimage.com

This book is a translation from the original published under ISBN 978-3-330-77256-4.

Publisher:
Sciencia Scripts
is a trademark of
Dodo Books Indian Ocean Ltd. and OmniScriptum S.R.L publishing group

120 High Road, East Finchley, London, N2 9ED, United Kingdom
Str. Armeneasca 28/1, office 1, Chisinau MD-2012, Republic of Moldova, Europe
Managing Directors: Ieva Konstantinova, Victoria Ursu
info@omniscriptum.com

Printed at: see last page
ISBN: 978-620-8-64302-7

SUMMARY

THE IMPACT OF NIGHT WORK ON NURSES' QUALITY OF LIFE:

A look at the men's team.

Rafael Lemes de Aquino

Author

Master's Degree in Environmental Health and Workers' Health from the Postgraduate Program in Environmental Health and Workers' Health - PPGAT/UFU (2017). Specialist in Occupational Nursing from Cândido Mendes University (2016). Degree in Geography - UFU (2014). MBA in Auditing and Forensics from FACI/UFU (2008). Bachelor's degree in Nursing from the University Center of the Triângulo Mineiro - UNITRI (2007).

Ailton de Souza Aragao

Co-author

PhD in Collective Health from the Ribeirao Preto School of Nursing, University of São Paulo (2011). Master in Sociology, UNESP, Araraquara, SP (2005), Bachelor in Social Sciences, UNESP, Marilia, SP (2001). Lecturer in the Postgraduate Program in Environmental Health and Workers' Health - PPGAT/UFU, Uberlândia, MG. Lecturer in Health and Society and Violence and Health at UFTM, Campus Uberaba, MG.

2017

I dedicate this work to the most precious and beautiful things in my life: my family, my friends and my cats. Especially to my mother Maria Regina Arantes Lemes and Aunt Neusa de Aquino (in memoriam) who, even though they were absent, I know they cheered me on and were fundamental to my formation and the realization of this dream.

"Your work will take up a large part of your life, and the only way to be truly satisfied is to do what you believe is a great job. And the only way to do a great job is to do what you love to do. If you haven't found it yet, keep looking... So work at it, face the difficult decisions, don't get carried away by emotion, be firm, seek information and don't make assumptions, seek help, stay focused and concentrate on what you're good at".

STEVE JOBS, 2009.

PREFACE

The book *Impacto do trabalho nocturno na qualidade* de *vida do Enfermeiro,* by Rafael Lemes de Aquino, is part of his master's thesis defended at the Postgraduate Program in Environmental Health and Workers' Health at the Federal University of Uberlândia, in August 2016.

This is a timely and necessary publication for academic debate and social practice, aimed at specific audiences interested both in gender issues and in the importance of the quality of life of the largest workforce of health professionals in Brazil and the world, nursing.

Man has been caring for man since before he was truly human. Caring for others changes from an instinctive act to a social one when it moves from the private to the public sphere. Thus, caring for the other, caring for one's neighbor, has changed scale and place throughout human history.

Since the advent of society within the human species, the cognitive abstraction that produces culture and religion in man has been reflected in the care of the sick, the needy and the elderly. Thus, caring for the other, for one's fellow man, moves from the close family or private sphere to the public sphere, when this care becomes the responsibility of a representative of the clan, tribe or social grouping, who are designated emissaries or spokespeople for the supernatural, for the entities of the metaphysical.

Shamans, shamans or healers began to play the role of caring for the sick and the elderly in ancient social groupings in various parts of the planet and, in some cases, even in present-day societies. However, slowly and progressively, in the area of health, scientific rationality is overcoming the supernatural. The care of the other in the public sphere is deepening, surpassing that of the family, and the place of care is moving from the home (private-family) to the specific (public).

From the Greek Latrioes, the Roman bath houses, the French Hotel-Dieu (from

650-656), the places chosen in China and Buddhist India, the houses of Mercy in Portugal (1498) and then Brazil, we arrive, as Foucault says, at the Hospitals of 19th century modernity. With this, the advent of the hospital, this model place for providing services to care for the sick in contemporary Western times, "contaminates" other societies around the world and becomes, in most cases, the "place" for caring for human illnesses.

To the same extent as the complexification of human care, in other words, in the area of public health, hospitals are aligning themselves with the transformations of human knowledge, academic knowledge impregnated by positivist rationalism and steeped in the ideas and ideals of the Enlightenment, the processes of secularization and standardization are gaining momentum.

Thus, to the same extent as this phenomenon, health professionals specialize and diversify. In the sphere of the specific, health professionals specialize to meet the needs of the new demands created by the complexification of contemporary human society, diversifying and breaking down prejudiced paradigms in the sphere of gender and work. Activities that were once designated as exclusive to one sex, such as nursing and midwifery, have taken on a new masculine and feminine profile. The professional category of nurses grows stronger, moves from the empirical to the scientific-academic and slowly incorporates men into its technical staff, as well as dividing and specializing into sub-areas.

And let there be light!

From the 19th century onwards, the science that underpins capitalism revolutionizes the night with electricity, as well as giving greater impetus to the driving force of capital. This advent was fundamental to understanding the expansion of the hours of caring for others.

Since the dawn of the human species, Homo Sapiens has been looking for ways and techniques to protect itself, to heal itself and to live in the absence of the natural and nurturing light of the sun. Natural sunlight has always been a blessing for the fragile human species, which had to protect itself from predators with better night vision than ours. Daylight was a consolation and a safeguard for those humans who had to take refuge in caves, holes and all sorts of places that were difficult to reach from the claws and eyes of nocturnal predators who had us for dinner.

The mastery of fire brought the human race an improvement in the intake of animal protein, which could now be better prepared and digested. In addition, the mastery of fire served to increase the protection of "homes" with better lighting. Whether caves, logs or holes, the illumination of fire has enabled us to improve our quality of life and increase the number of hours we can be alert with better vision. Unnatural lighting changes people's habits and human culture is produced in people's communal and then family "homes".

Artificial light has made the night brighter and more productive. It has shortened our sleep and stretched out our daily activities. Whether it's artificial lighting, produced by torches, burning oils or electricity, it revolutionizes, burns and disfigures the night and the darkness associated with it. The day grew longer. Night and the nocturnal have been shortened in line with technical advances in lighting.

As a result, lighting, however precarious, has made work and conversation everyday activities since ancient times. The family and clan circles of the early megalithic Homo sapiens relied on the light emitted from bonfires. Tools, weapons and clothes were produced in the same environment. This same image illustrates the environment of Neolithic houses with the fire burning in the center of the communal dwelling.

The dwellings of ancient man, from the Roman city to the Greek polis, were lit internally with lamparina-based fires and externally with torches or containers soaked in oils or bitumen. In the modern 19th century, with the advent of electricity and its consequent mechanical use, public and private night lighting was revolutionized and possibilities opened up that had never been imagined before.

The electricity technology of the modern era gives freedom to man and huge gains to the growing capitalist mode of production. This "new" source of energy generates radical interventions in the world of human work. From factories to hospitals, night shifts take away the exclusive "right" of capitalist work.

However, the human species was "designed" by evolution for daytime habits. Alert and awakening hormones are dumped into our bodies when bathed in natural light. With artificial light, this doesn't happen so easily. In the absence of sunlight, our body is flooded with melatonin. Melatonin is produced in the dark, i.e. at night, and its release begins as soon as we close our eyes.

When you wake up in the morning, your body stops releasing growth hormone (GH) and starts producing cortisol, which helps maintain emotional stability. In the process, it also releases TSH, Leptin, Ghrelin and INSULIN, among others. Cortisol is our "alarm clock" and its release peaks in the morning. When we don't sleep, its rhythm is altered and it can generate effects similar to stress (anxiety, excessive activity, etc.).

According to psychiatrist Maria Paz Loayza Hidalgo, from the Chronobiology Laboratory at the Hospital de Clinicas de Porto Alegre (HCPA), "people who work night shifts or are exposed to brightly lit environments at night are at greater risk of developing some types of cancer, depression and obesity. This is because artificial light stimuli confuse the body and contribute to a reduction in melatonin production."

Neurotransmitters such as serotonin are responsible for transmitting data between neurons and also for our brain's state of alertness. In order for a person to sleep properly, it acts in two different ways. At first, it regulates the first phase of sleep and for the deepest phase to take place - REM sleep - this neurotransmitter must be inhibited. The functions of this neurotransmitter go beyond communication between neurons. Heart rhythm, sleep, appetite and the regulation of certain hormones are all part of this substance's functions.

It is also responsible for a person's mood, body temperature, sensitivity to pain, movement and intellectual functions. Tryptophan is converted into serotonin, which is converted into melatonin. This is why the concentration of Serotonin is increased in the pineal gland during the day, when there is light, contrary to what happens with Melatonin.

The hormonal and neurotransmitter mechanisms of day and night, day and night, with and without natural light are still the subject of scientific study and academic debate. But advances in this area of knowledge allow us to make some pertinent observations. One of them is that night work is unnatural, stressful and low-yielding.

The night work of a professional whose job it is to be vigilant and pay extra attention is an even more stressful situation. Nursing is, in itself, a job full of adrenaline and stress factors. When the individual nursing professional is exposed to risks in their activities, such as in certain situations and places that exacerbate such risks, the "trigger" of stress unleashes serious health problems for this individual. The reality of the situation becomes clear. The mask of the health professional's invulnerability falls away. They expose what the individual nursing professional really is: homo *sapiens sapiens*.

In other words, it makes real what was intended to be theatrical: we are all human. Human beings. With their frailties, their anguish and all the ancestral burden of 300,000 years of evolutionary history.

Yes, we are human and we have our desires, fantasies, fears and needs, some socially acquired, and others, deeper, hidden in our hominid mind, which surface from time to time in this so-called modern society from small or large traumas, which can be derived from working night shifts, from the violence of the urban social fabric, from the individualistic and hypocritical nature of the human masses or even from the simple fact that society and work in globalized modernity are stressful.

Prof. Dr. Winston Kleiber de Almeida Bacelar

Coordinator Master's Degree in Environmental Health and Workers' Health-PPGAT/UFU **INSTITUTE OF GEOGRAPHY** Federal University of Uberlândia

PRESENTATION

At this point, I present my notes and their entire structure, containing the theoretical and methodological references, as well as the results and their discussion. It is worth mentioning that this work allows me to review important concepts and themes that are very present in my professional activity.

It is worth mentioning that in my academic and professional career, I sought to learn about the nursing profession through a vocational technical course, motivated by personal reasons, I initially took the nursing assistant course, then the nursing technician course, and during this period I empirically realized the low presence of men in the profession, something that has always caused personal concerns.

Believing that the presence of men in the profession was a great gain and contribution to day-to-day life and to de-characterizing a practice configured as feminine, another point worth mentioning was that over 15 years of work, I observed that the male presence was greater at night, a fact that was more evident when I graduated in nursing.

In addition, it is necessary to mention other observations that were made, such as: the majority of the nursing staff who worked and still work at night, regardless of their gender, do so because they have another job during the day, or because they have to look after children or elderly relatives, or in order to continue their studies.

It is important to emphasize that the work of the nursing team, which is present 24 hours a day, is the largest contingent of personnel in healthcare environments. And even though it is a mostly female profession, whether in the social, cultural and historical context, and due to the multiple perceptions during my professional career, I proposed to study and talk about the impacts of night workers on their quality of life, especially the male gender.

However, as much as the possibility of doing a professional master's degree can contribute to understanding some of the common and present consequences of everyday work, it goes much further, as it allows us to glimpse a reality that can reduce the damage and problems inherent in the work activity, in this case the men in the nursing team.

I work with issues related to gender, quality of life and night work because of my professional choice. When I chose nursing as a profession, I came across complex social relationships that are anchored in these issues, and the fact that a man works in a profession that is historically and culturally thought of and practiced mostly by women does not happen without the contribution and inclusion of the male figure in order to improve and perfect the profession.

I believe that my expectations in terms of acquiring new knowledge about Workers' Health and Environmental Health went far beyond what I initially expected, as it enabled me to gain information, exchange experiences and be able to multiply the theoretical teachings and reflections in my professional environment.

Another important point was the exchange between the students, and that even though it was a professional master's degree, its composition of numerous health and environmental professionals contributed greatly to the debates, enriching the daily interaction in the subjects taken by all.

Thus, research into the professional environment and its effects on the health of workers, especially nursing staff, has enabled a better understanding of situations and reality, in an attempt to create possibilities and actions to prevent the illnesses and problems inherent to the activity.

Facing up to this challenge was great, as it allowed me to have a better dialogue on how to apply the theoretical knowledge I had acquired to my professional practice. I believe that this was only possible because studying and understanding a subject that is present not only in my day-to-day life, but also in that of countless other professionals, helped me to seek improvements and answers to many possible problems of intervention and action.

In this way, it was possible to approach and deal with some themes to be analyzed, confronted and correlated such as the issue of Quality of Life; Work as a category of analysis; night work as the main focus of the study; Nursing as a science and profession and the issue of Gender, specifically men in a profession considered to be feminine.

In this sense, the aim of my master's research was to discuss, through an investigation, the impacts that night work has on the quality of life of male professionals, as well as to analyze, using a specific quality of life instrument, the main problems and damages inherent to this group of workers. It unfolds with some categories of analysis in an attempt to understand and discuss the theme through domains, be they physical, psychological, environmental, social relations and general, correlating with the overall quality of life and their perceptions of general health.

In view of this, do male nursing professionals, be they nurses, technicians or nursing assistants, who work night shifts suffer what kind of impact on their quality of life and health compared to other nursing workers on other shifts? What are the main obstacles and effects of the shift on their quality of life?

In addition to the introductory reflections and the important points highlighted, we also present some questions that guide the research process: in the midst of the specific legislation and its compliance, is there a possibility among the legal intricacies to better and more effectively promote the quality of life of nursing workers, especially those on the night shift?

We still have a lot of employees taking time off work, causing costs that could be avoided with preventive measures and health promotion. But is there any advantage in changing the way we look at things, whether it's organizational structures or the service routine itself, in order to minimize occupational illnesses and sick leave? Wouldn't hardship, unhealthiness and sleep deprivation alone be elements that deserve attention when we talk about quality of life?

These issues are very clear when compared with the recorded numbers of sick leaves and illnesses among health professionals, even though they are not exclusive to the nursing team, let alone the gender issue. In this way, scientific knowledge on workers' health has sought to explain the multiple dimensions between society, the environment and health.

Having presented the focus of my study, albeit briefly, I will now present the structure of the chapters that make up the dissertation. To begin with, in my presentation I will outline some of the points that led me to study gender relations in the profession over the course of my academic and professional career.

This is followed by an introduction to the work, contextualizing and bringing together the main themes that will be developed and addressed in the subsequent chapters, in an attempt to make some important inferences and reflections for the theoretical construction of this research.

In the first chapter, I outline the main guiding themes for the analysis of this work with some fragments of theoretical and conceptual frameworks on work, quality of life, nursing, gender and night work, with a view to understanding the context and delimitations of gender issues in the nursing profession.

In the next chapter, I present the fields covered by the study and the methodological paths I took to carry it out. In the methodological pathway, the proposed study is cross-sectional in nature with a quantitative approach, and with it I set out to examine the quality of life of male nursing staff who work at night using the WHOQOL-Abbreviated data collection instrument, an abbreviated quality of life assessment instrument developed by the World Health Organization (WHO) and adapted into Brazilian Portuguese.

I also describe the entire scenario of the study, present and define the methods of this instrument and all its regulations for the data collection process, as well as the data analysis procedures.

The final chapter presents the results and discussion of the data grouped by domains or analytical units generated from the application of the questionnaire with the male staff who work at night, in which I try to problematize the main findings, as well as making a comparison of the data focusing on the variables of the instrument with age, marital status, position, length of service and employment relationship. Finally, this is the path I intend to follow in the chapters that follow.

INTRODUCTION

The relationship that man has established with the environment has been shaped in various ways, both in its occupation and in living in society itself, which has had some significant impacts that deserve analysis and study.

Nowadays, one of the most wide-ranging and relevant issues is health, and concern about the environmental aspect and its relationship with man is essential for a better understanding of the reality we live in.

In this process, the theme of quality of life and workers' health plays an important role, since the social and environmental aspects of living in society are generally largely responsible for the problems that afflict the majority of the population.

This is not a recent concern, because this connection between the environment and countless illnesses has been made since ancient times. Therefore, it is in this context that environmental health and workers' health, as well as the health-disease process in professionals who deal exclusively with health recovery, are studied and approached from various angles in an attempt to minimize the damage caused by work activities, seeking ways to improve their quality of life.

Thus, in an attempt to understand the process surrounding these issues, such as work in its various shifts, especially the night shift and those performed by male professionals in the nursing team, we try to identify how the dynamics of the various social and economic factors that favor or not favor the emergence of illnesses work.

Based on the revealing data from a national study of the nursing category throughout our territory, entitled "Profile of Nursing in Brazil", where the Federal Nursing Council (COFEN) together with the Osvaldo Cruz Foundation (FIOCRUZ) surveyed a population of more than 1.8 million nursing professionals. It revealed important data such as the increase in male participation, registering a growing presence of 14.4% of men with a new trend towards the masculinization of the profession.

And even though nursing, by tradition, culture and historically, the data confirms the predominance of women, and that even after many decades the health sector is structurally female.

Among these ideas, this research is justified in view of the scarcity of studies that effectively delve into the theme of male night nursing workers in relation to their quality of life, which can be approached from a workers' health perspective.

However, it is well known how important it is to study a field that dialogues and approaches the professional and their professional activity, which is their work activity or shift, and thus be a guide for proposals to improve the promotion, prevention and identification of illnesses and diseases in the workplace.

In short, studying the relationships between work, health and the impact that night work has on the quality of life of professionals makes a lot of contributions to improving the many common problems encountered today.

1 THEORETICAL FRAMEWORK

This chapter deals with a review of the literature that sought aspects to support the research and promote a better understanding of the subject, helping to analyze the results. It addresses elements considered fundamental to understanding Quality of Life, Work, Nursing and Gender and Night Work.

The concern with knowledge of reality is a constant in human life, since research is a form of investigation that aims to find answers to society's questions through scientific procedures (BEUREN, 2004).

In the globalized world in which we live, Santos (2002, p.63) states that geographical space is gaining new attributes, important contours, new characteristics, new definitions and meanings. And also "a new importance, because the efficiency of actions is strictly related to their location, thus generating extreme competitiveness".

Lakatos (2010) cites that it is from the relationship that man has with the world, in his constant questioning and inquiry, in whatever field he is in, that awareness and knowledge of the reality of the experiences of his social group arise.

In this sense, Nolasco (2001) argues that in traditional societies, social recognition and visibility are defined according to hierarchies that articulate different subjects within the culture. This mesh cuts across different levels (class, gender, race and sexual choice), establishing values, subordinations and contexts between them.

However, it is worth highlighting the process of construction and understanding, which Gerard (1981) states is an analysis that makes it possible to observe the components of a whole, perceiving their possible relationships and moving from a key idea to a set of more specific ideas, going through generalization and finally to criticism.

Therefore, all scientific work is based on a theoretical framework, which supports it and gives it credibility and enriches it. This framework is characterized by bibliographic documentation, by scanning the literature through bibliographic research (MINEO, 2005).

1.1 WORK

Since the dawn of humanity, work has been used to produce life in the relationship between human beings and nature, creating use values to make their existence possible. And when we think about the historical evolution of work, Bauman (2001), presents an addendum, when talking about chronology and its countless historical innovations in living in society, we come across a modernity that begins when space and time are intimately separated from the practice of life and theorized through actions.

Since we are born into a group, we grow up in different groups and become adults participating in many other groups. Some remain with us throughout our lives, such as family and friends, while others become present at specific stages of our development (RODRIGUES, 2009).

Men are conditioned beings, because everything they come into contact with immediately becomes a condition of their existence, that is, in addition to the conditions under which life is given to man on Earth, they constantly create their own conditions (ARENDT, 2014).

Work is a fundamental condition of human existence. Rohm (2015) points out that through it, man relates to nature, constructs his reality, inserts himself into group contexts, acting in roles and ultimately promoting the perpetuation of his existence.

However, modern scientific thought has tended towards reduction, setting itself the challenge of achieving maximum precision and objectivity by translating events into abstract, calculable and demonstrable schemes (CZERESNIA, 2009).

In turn, globalization has brought new changes to work processes, so that the very meaning of work and employment has changed (PIGNATI et al., 2013).

Thus, the concepts of work process, worker, health and work-related illness structure the field and help to understand the social, economic, technological and organizational conditioning factors of the living and health conditions of the population and workers resulting from the development model adopted by the country (PINHEIRO et al., 2012).

Dejours (2004) categorically states that the act of working is not just a construction of reality from a raw material, but goes further. Working means transforming concrete reality, but also modifying psychic structures inherent to one's own subjectivity, which can sometimes serve as personal fulfillment, or even as an elaboration of frustrations.

Arendt (2014) organizes and systematizes the human condition into three aspects: labor, which is the biological process necessary for the survival of the individual and the human species; work, which is the activity that man has imposed on his own species as the result of a cultural process; and action, which is man's need to live among his peers, his nature being eminently social.

"In Portuguese, although there is labor and work, it is possible to find in the same word work both meanings: that of carrying out a work that expresses you, that gives you social recognition and remains beyond your lifetime; and that of routine and repetitive effort, without freedom, with consumable results and inevitable discomfort. In the dictionary, the first meaning appears to be the application of human forces and faculties to achieve a certain end; coordinated activity of a physical or intellectual nature, necessary for any task, service or undertaking; exercising this activity as a permanent occupation , trade, profession" (ALBORNOZ, 2008, p. 9).

It can be said that work at the moment is characterized by intensification, with high demand and requirements, little autonomy and control by the worker; diversity and complementarity within production chains; precariousness of social ties and protection, increasing the vulnerability of workers and environmental degradation and quality of life (PINHEIRO, et al., 2012).

Given its importance in human life and relationships, the ideal would be for the working environment to be as healthy as possible, a means for man to achieve maturity and autonomy as a social being (HORN; COTANDA, 2011).

In everyday language, the word work has many meanings. Although it seems understandable, as one of the basic forms of human action, its content fluctuates. Sometimes, charged with emotion, it recalls pain, torture, sweat on the face, fatigue, among other meanings (ALBORNOZ, 2008).

Because the role of work in the lives and health of individuals is fundamental insofar as we are aware of the harm that the conditions of the physical working environment can cause workers, whether it's occupational diseases or the work itself, or the accidents themselves, all of which attack the body of the worker (DEJOURS, 1986).

Albornoz (2008) reaffirms that work is not only a duty, but a right, because through it man is man, he makes himself, he appears, as he creates and enters into a relationship with others, with his time, creates his world, becomes recognized and leaves the mark of his passage on the planet on which he lives.

> If the transformation of human capital into qualifications is an operation of social judgment, this implies that it passes through the filter of social representations: those that differentiate work, tasks and professions, and also those that differentiate workers between them. In these operations of social judgment about work and workers, representations of masculinity and femininity occupy as central a place as representations of the capital-labor relationship (MARUANI, HIRATA, 2003, p. 69).

In the 18th century, an important event took place, the Industrial Revolution, and some phenomena arose as a result of the beginning of the industrialization process and the use of a mechanized work model. The "history of the realization of the social being is objectified through the production and reproduction of its existence, an act that takes place through work". It is through work, in its everydayness, that man becomes social, distinguishing himself from all non-human forms (ANTUNES, 2015, p.168).

By work relationships we mean all the human ties created by the work organization, whether they are relationships with the hierarchy, with managers, with supervisors, with other workers, and which are sometimes unpleasant, even unbearable, and generate conflicts within the team (DEJOURS, 2015).

In a society of individuals, everyone must be an individual. The members of such a society are anything but different and unique individuals. On the contrary, they are strictly similar to everyone else in that they have to follow the same life strategy and use common, commonly recognizable and legitimate symbols to convince others that they are doing so (BAUMAN, 2009).

Alves (2011) adds to the chronology of the contextualization of reproduction and development in the face of capitalism and its evolution by pointing out that capital's offensive is not restricted to the instance of production itself, but today, more than ever, under manipulative capitalism, it reaches instances of social reproduction, placed as organic nexuses of production as a social totality. In this way, it is through the ideological storm of values, expectations and market utopias that the new productive man of capital is sought to be formed.

Unlike in the animal world, where generations follow one another and are subjected to the same genetic program, in the human world each generation is faced with the enormous challenge of receiving its cultural heritage from the past, transforming it and projecting it into the future, carrying forward the process of civilization (REY, 2011).

Thus, some time after this revolution, the world went through a major crisis as a result of the stock market crash, and then needed to recreate means of production that could continue to sustain the machine of capitalism (ALVIM, 2006).

A practical example of this is the discourse developed during productive restructuring, which showed that the downgrading of women's work, even if attenuated in some companies, remained very clear in many others, both in Brazil and abroad. And due to the numerous asymmetries relating to gender and ethnicity, discrimination of various kinds persisted, despite the business discourses that emphasized overcoming inequalities and discrimination under participatory forms of management (SILVA, 2011).

It is important to know that the pattern of capitalist accumulation, in which societies and economies face a series of changes and problems such as the growth of unemployment and the lack of dignified conditions of survival for all citizens, forces us to rethink the model of economic development, presenting it as one of the greatest challenges of today's society.

With the advent of capitalism and the spread of the liberal model, which aimed to open up the market and consequently increase competitiveness, as well as the rise of technological globalization, the formula: liberal economy, globalized and competitive market, technological advance, speed in the transmission of information and commercialization of technology has led organizations to abandon the previous management model and start relying on people as a solution to obtain a competitive edge (ALVIM, 2006).

The productive changes that have surrounded the world and have been natural conditions of contemporaneity, even though they are victims of exacerbated globalization, are still shaped by old ideas and models. Sato (2002) corroborates this information and points out that there is still the archaic idea that work is directly linked to slavery.

As a result, Cavalcante (2014) points out that work is no longer just a repetitive form of reproduction, but has become more strategic in order to exceed targets. Marx (1985) sees work as something relational, where there is a relationship between man and nature, with man playing the role of a natural power, using the forces he is endowed with to shape the material into a form that is useful for life.

> [...] labor is a process between man and nature, a process in which man, by his own action,

mediates, regulates and controls his metabolism with nature. He himself confronts natural matter as a natural force (MARX, 1985, p.149).

However, it is important to note that work may not correspond to the needs and desires of individuals, nor may it offer the possibility of recognition or allow workers to express themselves freely. The individual doesn't recognize themselves in what they do and their work becomes meaningless (DEJOURS, 1992).

If we understand experience and history on planet Earth as a challenging and dynamic process of humanization, we will find ourselves facing the prospect of building work as a creative, autonomous and free activity (PIGNATI et al., 2013).

For Busetti (1998), we should see it as a whole, not just a mechanical assembly that is subject to possible repairs and, for this reason, take an integrated view of health and quality of life, in an attempt to address aspects that promote balance and human development in harmony.

There has been a growth in the topic of workers' health, because it shows that the risk situations present in work environments also modify the health pattern of the population in general, since a large contingent of this population is made up of workers themselves. And also because the production process can alter environmental conditions, i.e. ecological-social conditions, which influence the health of different human groups (ROUQUAYROL, 2003).

The concept of the human person is not restricted to the dimension of subjectivity (human subject with body and mind; or even psychic subject); but also implies the element of alterity (the other as neighbor and the dimension of sociability); and the element of individuality, where we have the social (class) individual human singularity, constituting its unique personality through processes of socialization/individualization (ALVES, 2014).

Thus, the human condition of work is life itself, because work is the activity that corresponds to the biological process of the human body, whose spontaneous growth, metabolism and resulting decline are linked to the vital needs produced and supplied to the vital process by work (ARENDT, 2014).

Alves (2014), when mentioning the social issue, states that an emancipated human society of self-organized producers, where human subjects have re-appropriated the objective and subjective conditions of social production (working and management conditions), the technical basis of the new informational machines, have contributed to the development of new human Virtualities, explaining a new way of organizing work and a new way of life.

The apparent benefits obtained by workers in the process of work are largely offset by capital, since the workers' need to think, act and propose must always take into account the company's intrinsic objectives, which are often masked by the need to meet the desires of the consumer market (ANTUNES, 2009).

The processes necessary for man to modify materials extracted from nature to transform them into useful products, in line with current technological needs, lead to the dispersion of substances in the workplace, most of which are harmful to health and the environment (LUONGO, 2012).

Thus, work ensures not only the survival of the individual, but "the life of the species, because the work and its product, a human artifact, give a measure of permanence and durability to the futility of mortal life and the ephemeral nature of human time" (ARENDT, 2014, p. 11).

Therefore, health and illness are ways in which life manifests itself. They correspond to singular and subjective experiences that cannot be fully recognized and signified by words. In medicine, health is considered to be the "normal" state of the human organism. Normality cannot be accurately determined due to the large number of factors, such as gender, age, profession, susceptibility, individuality, which interact in each person's organism (ROCHA, 2012).

Health is mentioned as an essential factor for human development; one of the fields of action proposed in the context of health promotion is the creation of favorable environments; sustainable development places the human being as the central agent in the process of defending the environment and has the increase in healthy and quality life expectancy as its main aspect (CZERESNIA, 2009).

On the other hand, Carvalho (2014) defines health as a worker's asset, an essential and fundamental condition for social interaction, inseparable from work. Thus, health, safety and quality of life are minimum requirements for maintaining productivity and product quality.

It should be noted that workers share with non-workers ways of getting sick and dying resulting from lifestyle, gender, age, genetic profile and environmental risk factors to which they are all exposed and live with (PINHEIRO et al., 2012).

The World Health Organization's (WHO) definition of health is "a state of complete physical and social well-being and not simply the absence of disease or infirmity", and although this concept does not match reality, it is the starting point for a holistic view of health. And this definition has provided clues as to which domains should be considered when assessing health, well-being and the broader concept of quality of life (FLECK, 2008).

In this way, Rey (2011) states that since culture is not a given of nature, but a social construction, this generational task is crossed both by tradition, the transmission of the past, and by creation, the challenges of the present, and the projection of expectations for the future.

Still on the importance of the aspect of representations, Rey (2011) ratifies that illness was circumscribed to a social representation which, supported by the dominant beliefs of medicine, extended to a system of institutionalized practices that led human beings to feel defenceless, insecure and incompetent in the face of illness and to see their capacity for discernment, decision and action in relation to their own illness taken away.

In view of this, work becomes one of the elements that most interfere with the conditions and quality of life of man and his health, since work is a natural necessity and a right of the individual guaranteed by the constitution. Although work was established with the emergence of humanity, the relationship between work and illness was practically ignored until a few dozen years ago (CARVALHO, 2014).

> For the Unified Health System (SUS), a worker is anyone who carries out an activity to support themselves or their family, regardless of whether they have a formal contract or not. Workers are those who receive a salary, are self-employed, public servants, cooperative workers, trainees, apprentices, small employers, those who are involuntarily out of the labor market, such as the unemployed and pensioners, and those who work helping another family member, even if they don't receive a salary. All of these people may have health problems caused by the work they do or have done (BRASIL, 2002, p. 3).

Carvalho (2014) mentions the necessary and important processes that contextualize issues by mentioning that industrialization and the consequent economic and social development bring many benefits to man, including improved health conditions and quality of life.

On the other hand, all the activities involved in this process, such as the production and storage of food, the production and generation of energy, the extraction of minerals, the manufacture of different products, the provision of services, including transportation, are generally associated with exposure to chemical, physical, biological, ergonomic or psychosocial agents capable of causing health problems not only for workers, but also for the population in general, as well as damage to the environment.

Freud (1976) lists some of the sources that cause suffering in individuals, such as supernatural power; the fragility of the body; the inadequacy of the adaptive norms of individuals' relationships, all of which are important points for analysis and observation.

This is what Rouquayrol (2013) points out when he mentions that the occurrence of problems that are characterized as aggravations or suffering and are defined as illness as opposed to health is inherent to life in society, and only by reference to this life. In other words, a given way of living and collective existence, representing a certain quality of social life, can be defined as transgressions, and therefore diseases, or adjustments and improvements, and therefore health.

The ILO (International Labor Organization) and the WHO have highlighted the close relationship between health and work. Since there have been changes in work processes due to economic crises and the restructuring of production systems, there has been a proportional increase in psychosocial risks at work (NEFFA, 2015).

Even so, these risks are at the root of psychiatric and mental illnesses caused by stress, harassment, burnout, verbal and physical violence, sexual abuse and, increasingly, the precarious nature of work. Epidemiological studies show that these illnesses are quickly somatized and lead to cardiovascular accidents, heart attacks and musculoskeletal disorders.

For the Ministry of Health (MS), precarious work is understood as work done without social protection for workers and public administration. Defining the concept of precariousness is a very complex task, as the risks are assumed by workers regardless of their employment relationship, which in turn requires other correlations with flexibilization and productive restructuring, issues that deserve to be reviewed (EBERHARDT et al., 2015).

Rohm and Lopes (2015) make us reflect on our social roles, arguing that each individual is a productive member of society and the organizations in which they live and they know that they cannot be a subject without confronting otherness, without being part of a collective, without contributing to the common good.

1.2 QUALITY OF LIFE

The subject of quality of life and its relationship with health professionals has been much highlighted and studied, and due to its importance it is necessary to address the numerous relationships and their effects on the various social fields, specifically the professionals in the nursing team.

In addition, due to the countless advances that medicine has brought, among other consequences, life expectancy has been extended over the last few centuries. However, diseases that used to be lethal have become curable, allowing greater control of their signs and symptoms or even slowing down their natural course (FLECK, 2008).

Seidl (2004) points out that in the health sector, interest in the concept of Quality of Life (QoL) is relatively recent and stems, in part, from the new paradigms that have influenced the sector's policies and practices in recent decades. And that the determinants and conditioning factors of the health-disease process are mostly multifactorial and complex.

Because we are living in a world that is increasingly fast-paced and constantly changing, whether in terms of the economy, globalization or modern technologies that make it possible to manage opportunities differently and improve the way companies enter the competitive market, in order to improve earnings and be more competitive.

In this context, we have professions that are essential, such as the health sector, which need to be uninterrupted, more specifically the work of the nursing team. However, little or no attention is paid to quality of life at work, and this becomes a conceptual background to the weaknesses and hardships we find in some professional activities.

Neri (2007) states that the emphasis on satisfaction and activity follows some tendencies to believe that the effects of variables on perceived well-being are mediated by other things of an internal and very personal nature, i.e. they are seen in different ways by each individual.

And by social well-being, Dejours (1996) defines it as the freedom to act individually and collectively on the organization of work, that is, on the content of work, the division of tasks, the division of men and the relationships they maintain with each other.

Quality of life is closely linked to standard of living, which in turn is defined as the quantity and quality of goods and services that someone normally consumes with a given income, and which rises or falls according to the fluctuations that occur in income levels. It presupposes the ability to make a cultural synthesis of all the elements that a given society considers to be its standard of comfort and well-being, and is therefore a social construction with cultural relativity, since it reflects the knowledge, experiences and values of individuals (MARTINS, 2008).

Concern about quality of life has been growing in recent years, gaining ground and reflecting on issues relating to groups of people and their localities.

Contrary to what it may seem, this concern with lifestyle is very old and originated with Socrates around 400 years BC. However, the term quality of life was mentioned for the first time in 1964 by Lyndon Johnson, then US president, when he stated that a nation cannot be measured by its financial flows, but by the quality of life provided to people (PEDROSO, PILATTI, 2010).

Ferreira (2012) analyses that the current context of globalization, characterized by the diffusion of new technologies, the circulation of ideas, the exchange of goods and services, as well as the growth in the movement of capital and financial flows, has a particular impact on workers and their health.

In this perspective, the term health and quality of life were presented as synonyms, but it is necessary to emphasize that the concept of quality of life transcends that of health, since there are several points of intersection between both variables (FLECK, 2008).

Before introducing the concept and its approaches, it is necessary to mention that the quality of life in countries is analyzed from the point of view of the HDI

- Human Development Index, which takes into account social groups reflecting the life expectancy of their population, longevity, education, purchasing power and standard of living.

For the WHO, the HDI is a way of measuring the quality of life in countries by comparing wealth, the quality of the literacy process, education, average life expectancy, birth and mortality rates, among others. But this index is a guideline for measuring the places or countries with the best living conditions and access to basic elements for maintaining life as a group.

In other words, the quality of life of a society, group or country is necessary for proposing interventions in health and sanitary policies, as well as being an indicator of the level of basic conditions that involve physical, mental, psychological and emotional well-being, such as family, health and other parameters that affect human life. It should be noted that QoL is different from standard of living, since standard of living is an average that quantifies the quality and quantity of goods and services that a given person or group can access.

According to Figure 1, the WHO in 2013 presented a map characterizing the HDI and QoL, as their indices are a general average common to each place in the world. An important aspect is that Brazil's HDI is one of the most different within its regions, but when this index is related to QoL, it is superior to many other countries.

Figure 1: Map of the Quality of Life in the World.

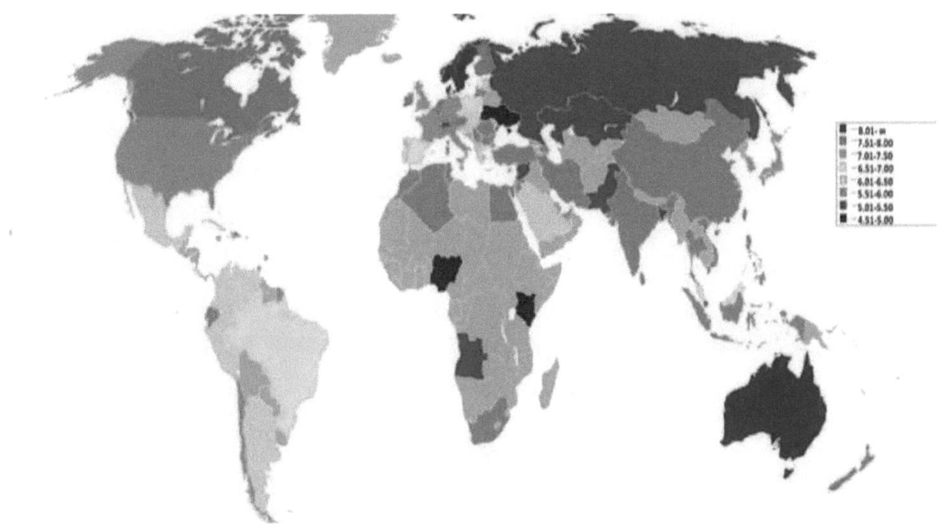

Source: WHO (2013).

Today, quality of life is defined by the World Health Organization (WHO) as "an individual's perception of his or her position in life, in the context of the culture and value system in which he or she lives and in relation to his or her goals, expectations, standards and concerns" (DINIZ, 2013).

The concept of quality of life was introduced into medicine at a time when traditional medical outcomes such as mortality and morbidity were being criticized for having too narrow a focus and failing to represent a large number of other potential outcomes (FLECK, 2008).

According to Chiavenato (2008), it involves creating, maintaining and improving the quality of work in its physical, psychological and social conditions, even if the market stimulates ample competition, becoming more concerned with profits and demanding more results and hours worked in the workplace from employees, as opposed to other concerns that do not promote QoL, such as the physical and mental health of its employees.

Diniz (2013) defines quality of life as a term that is complex to conceptualize and that over the last few decades there have been numerous scientists, philosophers, politicians and specialists from very different fields who have tried and are still trying to establish a consensus on this concept.

The term quality of life is the end result of a process of historical development whose first conceptual attempts emerged in 384 BC, when Aristotle referred to the association between "happiness" and "well-being". From the 20th century onwards, the expression "quality of life" became familiar, initially being used in common sense, informally, based on intuitive knowledge, devoid of definitions or scientific demarcations (BLAY; MARCHESONI; 2013, p.21).

Therefore, discussing and trying to understand themes and their consequences in health practice and even in concepts at different times leads us to reflect. We can conceptualize quality of life as something given to the individual, that is, singular, subjective and that differs only from having money to carry out one's activities, or even put it as a synonym for quantity of life.

Although there are countless definitions of QoL, it is necessary to understand that the concept is used in different ways, depending on the context in which it is presented. QoL can be seen as the opposite of quantity of life, length of life or even longevity, but it can also be seen as a synonym for the overall experience lived by an individual and their living conditions, including their health (FLECK, 2008).

We believe it is much broader, as it is directly related to other contexts besides health, well-being and happiness. It is directly related to the question of time, how each person is using it and employing what is necessary in their daily activities.

History and paleontology, for example, provide countless proofs that, since ancient times, people have sought to develop artifacts, tools and methods to minimize the wear and tear of work and make it more enjoyable (SANTANNA, 2011).

QoL, being a very complex and comprehensive term, does not have a pre-established concept and is often associated with both individual factors and the socio-environmental factors that surround the individual within a socio-cultural context. Given this complexity of meanings, various instruments have been developed to measure it, as their use facilitates knowledge of the needs of individuals in their specific life contexts (ANGELIM, et al., 2015).

The subject of quality of life at work or work-related quality of life (WQoL) is not the exclusive concern of today's researchers. In fact, since the dawn of civilization, man has been looking for ways to ease his struggle for survival. This concept has a direct impact on the job market, as it means measuring the level of satisfaction of the professional in comparison to the job they do in a particular place.

Thus, knowing the degree of relevance of the quality of life at work and its impacts that night work can generate for the worker makes it necessary to carry out studies that allow us to identify which factors affect the quality of life of night workers in the workplace and in their social life (ABREU, 2012).

Ferreira (2012) states that QWL is not only determined by individual characteristics (needs, values and expectations) or even situational ones (organizational structure, internal policies, technology), but above all by the systemic action of these with some factors such as: the possibility of recognition for results, the possibility of participating, the human relationship within the group and organization, as well as having a psychological and physical work environment that is minimally harmful to workers.

For these reasons, the WHO has taken the initiative with a collaborative project in its multicenter centers to develop a generic questionnaire widely used in various studies, which can be used in different groups focusing on their particularities and specificities.

The WHOQOL (Word Health Organization Quality of Life). In its original version, it consists of 100 questions distributed over six domains (physical, psychological, social relations, environment, spirituality and general) summed up by 100 specific facets, where the answers to the questions are given on a Likert-type scale (FLECK, 2008).

There are various QoL questionnaires, which can be generic or specific. The former are aimed at a general assessment of the life and health aspects of individuals who are ill or not, while the specific ones assess the particularities of a disease or condition, quantifying the impact of treatment and the health gains obtained.

Currently, the WHOQOL comes in original and abbreviated versions and can be found in more than 40 different languages, including Portuguese. This reflects not only the good acceptance of the instrument but also the growing interest in the subject in different scenarios, especially in the health area (ANGELIM, et al., 2015).

Table 1. WHOQOL-BREF instrument - the domains and facets of quality of life.

Domain	**Facets within domains**
1. Physical	Pain and discomfort Energy and fatigue Sleep and rest Mobility Activities of daily life Dependence on medication and treatments Work capacity
2. Psychological	Positive feelings Self-esteem Thinking, learning, memory and concentration Body image and appearance Negative feelings Spirituality/religion/personal beliefs
3. Social Relations	Personal relationships Social support Sexual activity
4. Environment	Physical security and protection Financial resources Physical Home environment environment Transportation

	Health and social care Opportunity to acquire new information Recreation and leisure
5. General	Overall quality of life and general health perceptions

Source: Fleck (2008).

The WHOQOL-BREF, or abbreviated version in Portuguese, has 26 questions relating to general QoL and general perception of health, which are divided into four domains (physical, psychological, social relations and environment) and 24 facets, each containing just one question, which are grouped into values on a scale of 0 to 100, measured in percentages (FLECK, 2008).

The need for short instruments that require little time to complete, while maintaining their validity, measurement and psychometric characteristics, has contributed to their use in different study groups.

Measuring subjective variables is not a simple task, as the choice of evaluation instrument is a process that requires a high level of subjectivity and that is supported by a series of normative and psychometric criteria (PEDROSO; PILATTI, 2010).

Kimura and Carandina (2009) state that even with all the applicability of this instrument, there is still a lack of instruments to measure the quality of life at work of health professionals and that take into account the specific nature of their professional activity.

1.3 GENDER

In recent decades, the history of workers has been rewritten at the same speed as global transformations, especially social and economic ones, as well as technological and scientific advances and demographic and income distribution changes, among other relevant factors, and constant adaptations have been demanded of them. As a result, the world of work is suffering the impacts of increasingly urgent and brief economic, political and social needs (HORN; COTANDA, 2011).

Throughout the historical process, work has taken many forms in order to meet the needs of each moment. However, it always remains a moment in which social relations come into being, with a view to social production and the reproduction of humanity (NOGUEIRA, 2011).

Looking back in time, Nolasco (2001) states that the Industrial Revolution established a format for working relationships that was problematized at the end of the 19th century amid a climate of hope and progress. And this phenomenon in the public sphere led to a series of changes in the private world, including the family and the relationship between men and women.

The analysis of work situations related to gender allows us to make specific proposals to improve these situations, aiming at changes and incidents in these socially imposed differences in female and male identities, which lead to the structuring of a discriminated labor market, with a negative impact on the health and lives of men and women (ANDRADE, 1997).

Thus, it is important to present the issue of gender within the professions and in this context Costa (2008) points out that the world of work, regardless of the organizational environment, is not always seen as the worker, since it is permeated by various segregations and discrimination of all kinds.

However, Melo (1986) points out that the organization of health services, in which nursing practice takes place, has been reflected in the dominant mode of production, encompassing social and professional categories, by capitalism.

The mission of nursing professionals is to care for the person, family and community in an integral way, considering the physical, psychosocial and spiritual dimensions. The act of caring is a skill that requires dedication, sensitivity, scientific knowledge, with mastery of concepts, techniques and work routines (OLIVEIRA, 2016).

In this sense, Haber (2001), ratifies that the health care environment is changing at an unprecedented pace and that nurses have the challenge of establishing their area of practice more comfortably and offering new critical approaches to deal with new and old problems to make a difference in the state of health.

For Marx, "the essence of human beings lies in their work. What they produce is what they are. Man is what he does. And the nature of individuals therefore depends on the material conditions that determine their productive activity" (ALBORNOZ, 2008, p.28).

As men live in communities, sharing a space at a particular time, social reproduction also implies the reproduction of a second domain, that of the ecological relations of the groups in which these communities are constituted (BARATA, 2009).

The act of working is directly linked to the relationship of production and reward, but it is also equipped with physical, psychological and emotional conditions. Neffa (2015) mentions that all work, even slave labor, requires the individual to have some energy to carry it out, making some parallels: "the dead don't work", since "work is the result of a voluntary human activity carried out under tension".

The nurse, or nursing professional, is in an unfavorable position, and can benefit little from their professional status to master their suffering or even transform it into something creative and spontaneous. However, in the opposite case, mobility, when present as a form of unconscious transference, allows for a huge mobilization of commitment and reflexive capacities (ROHM, 2015).

It is sometimes perceived that work becomes a fleeting way of compensating for unsatisfactory family relationships, directed to a greater extent at marital relationships and parent-child interactions. In this case, it's not difficult to see an affective or even accentuated disposition, as a way of compensating for the problems of private life, being projected into the hospital environment, as well as into the relationships established with the team (SILVA, 2011).

Work is not a category isolated from the productive and relational context. It gains an active dimension in reality from the actions of the subjects and is structured not as an act frozen in space and time, but as a dynamic process, which changes permeated by many interests, as many as the subjects who interact in the activity in which the daily labor around the production of care takes place (BARROS, 2016, p.16).

Thus, when it is assumed that a job requires an intense human relationship and interrelationship and bonding are essential, nursing work and health work are a productive action and social interaction (BARROS, 2015).

Nolasco (2001) and Bourdieu (2010) state that the crisis of the modern world has precipitated another model of society which is no longer standardized by tradition but by politics, law, technology and the market. Moreover, the old structures of the sexual division of labor still seem to determine the direction and form of changes, whether in jobs or careers that are more or less strongly gendered.

And faced with this universe of various themes and correlations with the professional activity of nursing, we are confronted with the subjectivity present at work, such as the sexual division of labor.

This is defined by Hirata (2002) as a generic term that refers to a whole series of social relations and the division of labor between the sexes refers to the male/female social relation, which crosses and is crossed by the other modalities of the social division of labor.

Historically, the representation of men does not correspond to what has been considered the masculine question for centuries, the basis for the conception of the different social representations of the subject. In the past it was necessary to hunt, war, fight and be feared, this was considered an evolutionary challenge.

However, these attributions no longer correspond to what is evolutionarily required of a man. Men's relationship with their bodies, their representation of themselves and their use of physical strength and gender have changed (NOLASCO, 2001).

Most discussions about gender in society emphasize a dichotomy. Starting from a biological division between men and women, gender is defined as social or psychological differences that correspond to this division, being built on it or caused by it (CONNELL, 2015).

In the case of health professionals, the social and emotional problem is multiplied, since most of their activities are carried out by women, who are generally more active in domestic life (HORN; COTANDA, 2011).

Inequality in the sexual division of labor in the productive and reproductive spheres is therefore central to power relations, especially the power exercised by men over women in the patriarchal family structure (NOGUEIRA, 2011).

The human body is an object of various meanings, whether social or cultural, attributed to it throughout human history. And these meanings refer to the patterns of interpretations about men and women in the contexts of the societies in which they settle and live in a given space and time.

According to Foucault (2014), these issues were described as the male body signifying strength and determination and the female body as fragility and protection. And for him, the body is a place of social control, because bodies are trained, shaped by the predominant historical forms of individuality, desire, masculinity and femininity.

In Portuguese, the word "genre" has various meanings depending on the field of knowledge in which it is used. However, in general terms, genus means a group of beings or objects that have the same origin or are linked by the similarity of one or more particularities. In biology, the term refers to the taxonomic category that groups together phylogenetically related species, distinguished from others by striking characteristics that allow them to be subdivided into families. In grammar, gender refers to classes of words that make it possible to establish the contrast between masculine and feminine, not always referring to differences in sex (BARATA, 2009, p. 73).

One of the strong expressions of this system that determines inequalities in social relations between the sexes is the sexual division of labor. The sexual division of labor is closely related to the capitalist mode of production and reproduction, fundamentally because it ensures greater profits for capital (CISNE, 2012).

The division between the sexes seems to be "in the order of things", as is sometimes said of what is normal, natural, to the point of being inevitable: it is present, at the same time as being objectified in things, in every social world (BOURDIEU, 2010).

Barata (2009) states that gender is not synonymous with sex, because in biology and also in the medical field, sex is just a marker of biological differences between individuals of the human species, which is related to the anatomical and physiological aspects of the reproductive system.

On the other hand, Bourdieu (2002) defines gender as a hierarchical social organization of sexual differences, which can be understood as a field that generates specific and complex social relations, in which men exercise their practices on a daily basis, showing a certain disposition towards social behavior.

Yet gender can also be seen as a central dimension of personal life, social relations and culture. "It is an arena in which we face difficult practical questions concerning justice, identity and even survival" (CONNELL, 2015, p.25).

However, gender is a serious trend in production, as the equality or supremacy of skills established by school is broken down by the rigidity of work organization. However, this rigidity is less and less justified by the technical characteristics of positions and jobs (MARUANI; HIRATA, 2003).

In everyday life, we take gender for granted and come to recognize a person as male or female, boy or girl, instantly and that these arrangements are so familiar that they seem to be part of our nature (CONNELL, 2015).

The construction of gender as an analytical category certainly has to do with the impasses of patriarchal theory and Marxist analysis, as much as with the autonomous development of psychoanalytical approaches. What is certain is that the axis of reflection in feminist research has become much more the search for the meanings of the representations of the feminine and the masculine, the cultural and historical constructions of gender relations (LOBO, 1991).

The relationship between gender and class allows us to see that in the universe of the productive and reproductive world, we also experience the realization of a gendered social construction, where men and women who work are, from family and school, differently qualified and trained to enter the labor market. And capitalism has been able to unequally appropriate this sexual division of labor (ANTUNES, 2009, p. 109).

When we talk about equality or inequality, we are comparing situations, without necessarily assigning a value judgment to what is equal or unequal. Fortunately, individuals and social groups have great differences and variability with regard to many characteristics, which is what makes life so interesting (BARATA, 2009).

The boundaries of masculinity and femininity are relatively mobile and depend to some extent on the demands of the production system in each historical period. However, capital itself is opposed to a more or less rigid total mobility of sexual attributes between sectors, sections and positions.

One of the reasons for this professional segregation is hypothetically the need to create a situation of incompatibility between female and male functions within companies, thus avoiding demands for equality (HAAG, 2001).

Today, the world is faced with urgent problems related to gender. Indeed, we see a new domain emerging in gender politics, with sharp questions about human rights, injustice, the global economy, environmental change, intergenerational relations, violence and the conditions for good living (CONNELL, 2015).

Even though nursing is a male-dominated profession, it has seen a greater number of women in its ranks and in the job market. In this circumstance, it would not be difficult to see the multiplicity of roles that women play in social life and which need to be articulated with professional life.

However, the traditional use of the concept of "sex" does not allow for the observation of historically constructed differences between men and women, while the use of the category of "gender" presupposes that differences in conditions lead to an unequal and hierarchical social structure that must be changed. It also overcomes the view that gender differences are eliminated within the workplace and allows us to look beyond bodily differences, the only parameter used by occupational medicine (ANDRADE, 1997).

Cisne (2012) points out that the existence of activities, professions and even skills considered feminine or masculine are not the result of a spontaneous or natural process. On the contrary, they result from the concrete construction of social relations which, in turn, are determined by the dominant interests of the prevailing social system, in this case, the capitalist patriarchy.

In many countries, women are the main agents of health, playing a fundamental role as factors of biopsychosocial well-being in the family, community and official health systems (ANDRADE, 1997).

Traditional societies have long maintained and those that survive today still seek to maintain a harmonious working relationship, whether with nature, in the transformation they make of it, or between the men and women who work and consume (PIGNATI et al., 2013).

Women are supposed to have one set of characteristics and men another. Women are caring, influential, communicative, emotional, intuitive and sexually loyal; men are aggressive, inflexible, taciturn, rational, analytical and promiscuous. These ideas have been widespread in European cultures since the 19th century, when the belief that women have a weaker intellect and less decision-making capacity than men was used to justify their exclusion from universities and the right to vote (CONNELL, 2015, p.111).

The biological difference between the sexes, i.e. between the male body and the female body, and specifically the anatomical difference between the sex organs, can thus be seen as a natural justification for the socially constructed difference between the sexes and especially for the social division of labor (BOURDIEU, 2010).

Nardi (2013) comments that gender relations, understood as the result of the processes of social construction of masculinity and femininity in a given society, are directly implicated in the ways in which not only gender relations are structured, but also work relations, public health policies, education, security, justice, assistance, in short, any and all social relations.

Studies carried out on the number of men and women in the nursing profession in the 1980s found a 94% female predominance. In the most recent survey, in which the Profile of Brazilian Nursing was drawn up in 2013 by the Federal Nursing Council (COFEN) and the Osvaldo Cruz Foundation (FIOCRUZ), among the more than 1.8 million professionals, male representation reached 15%, suggesting a masculinization of the nursing workforce.

Lopes (2005) reflects on the need to consider the historical influence of Florence Nightingale in institutionalizing nursing in England in 1862 as a profession for women, for which they are naturally prepared, based on values that were considered feminine. And that throughout the process of professionalization, these values and attributes will be exploited differently in institutionalized work.

On the other hand, during this period, several authors point out the male presence in nursing and that historically nursing was considered a male occupation in times of war, epidemics or calamities, which were important milestones for the evolution of nursing as a profession.

Even so, we can say that this male participation took a variety of forms, either religious men driven by devotion and charity, or military men driven by obedience to superior orders, or by war needs, or even doctors in search of assistants for their work (OGUISSO, 2007).

Costa (2010) highlights the importance of this cultural aspect found in care, which may have a strong influence on the maintenance of the male figure in nursing to treat patients of the same sex. Still following this idea, Vitorino (2012) questions the emergence of men in the nursing profession, when analyzing the history over the centuries, it is possible to find data that contradicts the myth that the category is "typically female", as it has been a field dominated by men for most of human history.

It should be noted that the presence and appropriation of men in the field of nursing was initially in certain areas of activity such as psychiatry, orthopedics and urology, and that these issues depended on the period and historical moment for their expansion in practice, since the image of the professional can be understood as a network of meanings and social representations exclusive to a particular profession (PEREIRA, 2011).

Torres (2004) mentions that nursing courses only accepted women students and that it was only in 1968, twenty-three years after the Second World War, with the unified entrance exam after the university reform, that the first practical nurses for the army and military police emerged.

The large number of women in nursing compared to men, in addition to the well-known historical roots of women, is probably also due to the fact that the population of women is higher than that of men, with 52% women to 48% men according to IBGE data in 2015.

Barbosa (2009) states that it is extremely interesting that in wars, men only became nurses when they were considered unfit to perform another function, which for many was a form of punishment.

On the other hand, we also have the issue that these professionals face a lot, the prejudice that exists in their own social context, often having their own sexual orientation questioned, ending up encountering some obstacles in the professional relationship, within the team and with the user.

For Silva (2012), we need to bear in mind that the context in which men and women live is not the result of biological destiny, as historically tried to be assumed, but rather comes from social constructions. And that, therefore, they form two social groups that are engaged in a specific relationship, and this relationship has a material basis which is work, and this is revealed through the social division of labor between the sexes.

The term "sexual division of labor" applies to new configurations with different contents, as it is a sociographic term which studies the differential distribution of men and women in the labor market, in their trades and professions and the variables in time and space of this distribution (HIRATA et al., 2007).

However, Souza (2014) explains that sexist divisions are present and clearly visible within the nursing profession, and that although men have gained ground within the profession, there is still a certain resistance to the presence of men in some types of practice developed by these professionals.

1.4 NURSING

The profession arose from the development and evolution of health practices over the course of historical periods. At an early stage of civilization, health actions guaranteed man's survival, as well as being associated with women's work (GEOVANINI, 1995).

Oliveira (1997) states that nursing has been recognized as a high-risk occupation with particular health problems. However, the health risks arising during nurses' paid work cannot be attributed to a single tail, but rather to a set of factors present in the working environment.

From a historical point of view, Nursing is an area of knowledge that is increasingly developing nationally and internationally, due to the breadth and interdisciplinarity of its historical studies (FILHO, 2016).

When we think of the historical trajectory, the oldest reference is the organization proposed by Florence Nightingale, in 1854, in her role in the Crimean War and the various achievements attributed to her, which led her to be considered a precursor of modern nursing (BARROS, 2015).

On the other hand, Melo (2013) adds that nursing models emerged around the end of the 19th century, based on assumptions propagated by Nightingale, who aimed not only at technical formalization, but also at the inclusion of women in medical fields, based on maternal characteristics "inherent to all women", based on scientific knowledge, leaving aside religious and unrealistic convictions.

The relationship between the nursing profession and society brings with it concepts established during the historical trajectory of nursing, which has been influenced by the characteristics of the people who, for centuries, have exercised or exercised the activity linked to care (FILHO, 2016).

As for the professional practice of nursing activities, they are observed and regulated by Law 7498 of June 25, 1986, and the nursing team, respecting the degrees of qualification we have: the nurse; the nursing technician; the nursing assistant and midwife. It is important to note that each member of the team has skills, actions and competencies that are unique to their activity (COREN/MG, 2015).

Art. 8 - Nurses are responsible for: directing the nursing department that is part of the basic structure of the health institution, whether public or private, and heading up nursing services and units; organizing and directing nursing services and their technical and auxiliary activities in companies that provide these services; planning, organizing, coordinating, executing and evaluating nursing care services; direct nursing care for serious, life-threatening patients;

Art. 10 - The Nursing Technician performs auxiliary activities, at a medium technical level, assigned to the Nursing team, and is responsible for: assisting the Nurse in planning, programming, guiding and supervising Nursing care activities;

Art. 11 - The Nursing Assistant carries out medium-level auxiliary activities assigned to the Nursing team, and is responsible for: preparing patients for consultations, examinations and treatments; observing, recognizing and describing signs and symptoms, at the level of their qualification; carrying out specifically prescribed or routine treatments, in addition to other Nursing activities;

Art. 12 - The Midwife is responsible for: caring for the pregnant woman and the parturient; assisting normal childbirth, including at home; and caring for the puerperal woman and the newborn.

Paragraph Five - The activities referred to in this article are carried out under the supervision of an Obstetric Nurse, when carried out in health institutions, and, whenever possible, under the control and supervision of a health unit, when carried out at home or wherever necessary.

Art. 13 - The activities listed in arts. 10 and 11 can only be carried out under the supervision, guidance and direction of a nurse (COREN/MG, 2015, p. 27-32).

Since nursing is a profession that strives to care for and value the lives of others, it is essential that the team is provided with the best material and technical conditions and, above all, is committed to promoting the health of the team. Since work is always surrounded by disparate feelings influenced by environmental and social conditions and, most importantly, by the relationships established between team members (NEFFA, 2015).

When we think of the nursing world, we have the idea of a profession full of care and affection for those who are in a vulnerable or even debilitated condition. Therefore, the nursing worker is immersed in environmental and personal variables that require individual and collective coping, given that their subjectivity was built well before they were trained.

The dimension of job satisfaction in the nursing team is due to the intersubjective relationships that take place between members and their hierarchies, based on relationships of exchange and gain, rewards, salaries and promotions. But above all in minimizing individual suffering, which will be reflected in the group relationship, strengthened or unstable based on the bonds established between group members (ROLIM, 2013).

These teams generally spend their entire working hours immersed in the natural pressures of hospitals, such as emergency situations, infections, violence, night work, chemical agents and others. There is a mental and physical overload, increasing the possibility of errors and accidents for the professional.

The worker's health-disease process is the result of the set of conditions in which workers live, work and relate socially in their daily lives. Thus, due to unhealthy conditions, it is possible to say that they offer the opportunity for the appearance of diseases, whether occupational or not, or even the debilitation of the worker or the shortening of their useful or working life due to the aggressiveness to which they are subjected (CARVALHO, 2001).

Since the dawn of time, we can say that man has known and been the victim, most of the time fatally, of the risks existing in his work or activity. Speaking of the workplace, Bulhões (1998) points out that occupational risks can be hidden or even present in the workplace, whether due to ignorance, lack of knowledge or information, so that workers don't even suspect they exist. Work activities, in the production of a good or service, require a minimum amount of physical space to be carried out.

Luongo (2012) argues that the space is the work environment, which as a physical environment suffers interference of various kinds: physical, chemical, ergonomic and biological, which can be variables that compromise the performance of the activities carried out and need to be controlled, because in addition to interrupting work functions, they can cause harm to workers (LUONGO, 2012).

Carvalho (2001) discusses the recognition of risks and defines that it is necessary to carry out a detailed survey of information and data on the work environment in order to identify the existing agents, the potential risks associated with them and the priority for evaluation and control of this work environment.

The risks are associated with working conditions, in particular their organization and the nature or content of the activity, and specifically with the psychological content. For this reason, the "harm profile" of nursing is characterized by the following components:

Overstrain injuries, especially in the lumbar region, as a result of the physical effort involved in handling patients; reproductive damage and miscarriages; infections due to contact with patients and other biological agents (hospital infections); physical illnesses (contact dermatitis due to biological, physical and chemical agents is often found); minor accidents; physical aggression; alteration of the sleep-wake cycle, sleep disorders, headaches, gastrointestinal problems, eating disorders and others associated with the rotating work system (day-night); mental fatigue and emotional tension associated with stress, expressed in symptoms of anxiety, anguish or depression (OLIVEIRA, 1997, p. 120).120).

Considering that in their work some professionals, specifically health professionals, constantly deal with human fragility, pain, death, horror, the demands and pressures for assertiveness, speed and risk inherent in health work, they experience pleasure and suffering in their daily lives.

The current division of labor that we find today is a structure of work in shifts, which is no longer a priority for services such as health and safety, especially in industrialized countries, and countless other services have started to maintain the continuity of their production, at all times, during all 24 hours of the day (MARTINO, 2005).

In Brazil, nursing professionals are known to work long hours, with 12-hour shifts followed by 36 or 60 hours of rest. Long working hours can lead to exhaustion and fatigue, which can affect patient care (SILVA, ROTENBERG, FISCHER, 2011).

Shift work stems from the need to provide 24-hour services to companies and consumers, and is usually divided into three 8-hour shifts or two 12-hour shifts, every 24 hours, depending on people's ability to perform their duties (ABREU, 2012).

Bulhoes (1998, p.51) lists the unhealthy and arduous activities inherent in the nursing profession:

> Nursing workers are particularly vulnerable due to some of their own characteristics, including the fact that nursing is the largest single group of health professionals; that it provides round-the-clock care, 24 hours a day; that it is responsible for carrying out around 60% of health actions; that it is the category that comes into most physical contact with patients; that it is a female profession par excellence; and that it is very diverse in its training.

The mental stress generated in the hospital environment plays an important role in accidents at work, since it is involved in cognitive and affective factors. Generally speaking, mental overload affects attention, memory, reasoning and decision-making in extreme situations.

Following this idea, Bouyer (2015) ratifies that the suffering perceived at work is always a social suffering, as entire collectives are subjected to the exaggerated demands of exceeding high production targets.

Environmental risks are innumerable because they are physical, chemical and biological agents in the workplace which, depending on their nature, concentration or intensity and exposure time, are capable of causing damage to workers' health regardless of the location (MIRANDA, 1998).

In order to explain the differences in the occupational profiles of illness and death between men and women, it is necessary to refer to the gender condition, since this category makes it possible to explain specific situations in working life: incorporation into the labor market, discrimination, double working hours - paid and domestic work, tasks added to jobs. These aspects influence health, generating problems such as the higher frequency of accidents and musculoskeletal disorders among men and the higher number of unspecific illnesses among women (ANDRADE, 1997).

In carrying out their duties and functions, nursing staff are faced with conditions in which they are exposed to overloads and underloads, which generate various processes of wear and tear on the worker's body, be they physical, chemical, biological, mechanical, physiological and psychic.

Karino (2015) states that nursing professionals in the health sector are the most susceptible to accidents in the workplace due to the activities they carry out when providing care to patients.

Boyer (2015) ratifies that due to the various forms of work organization, this mode can lead workers to suffering and illness. Alarmingly, Collucci (2015) points out that more than 70% of nurses in the country do not feel safe in the workplace, and more than a fifth of workers report the existence of violence, especially psychological violence.

When we talk about the harmful effects and consequences on the health of these professionals when it comes to work engagement and well-being, it's important to know more about what professional burnout or even Burnolt syndrome is. Burnout is understood as something extremely related to working conditions, the response to which triggers a prolonged and chronic state of work-related stress characterized by exhaustion, emotional exhaustion, dehumanization, depersonalization and reduced personal accomplishment at work (CAVALCANTE et al., 2014).

On the other hand, a European study carried out in nine countries with nursing staff showed that the shift work carried out by these professionals is very harmful, and that due to sick leave there is a need to work overtime to maintain the service. The result was that the more overtime these professionals work, the higher the mortality rate in institutions, reaching 20% (LINDA et al. 2014).

Novaretti et al. (2014), following this theme, show that work overload related to the disproportion between the number of nursing professionals and patients is reported to be a risk factor for the increased incidence of hospital infections, adverse events, harm to patients and professionals, increasing the risk of hospital mortality.

The shortage of nursing workers in institutions means that the pace of work is intensified and, therefore, wear and tear. The WHO recommends a ratio of two nurses/1000 inhabitants, but despite the large contingent of nursing workers in the country, which according to COFEN data totals around 1.8 million workers, this is still a difficult number to reach due to regional differences and concentrations (FELLI, 2012).

Nogueira (2014) associates the changes that have taken place over the last 30 years in the world of work with the significant increase in the number of workers suffering from repetitive strain injuries and work-related musculoskeletal disorders (RSI/WMSDs). He lists some factors as the cause, such as: the increase in hours worked, the loss of labour rights, the acceleration in the pace of work, precariousness and changes in organizations and the mode of production.

A profession perceived as feminine or masculine is nothing more than the result of the sexual division of labor which, in turn, not only fosters inequalities between men and women, but also serves the dominant interests of a patriarchal capitalist society, especially through the overexploitation of so-called women's work (CISNE, 2012).

Each social practice is part of the world of work in a specific way. Thus, nursing work finds its professional activity in the tertiary sector of the economy, in the provision of health services (FELLI, 2015).

Understanding the relationship between technological knowledge, qualification and the new flexibility of work organization cannot do without incorporating the sexual division of labour into the analysis, in order to grasp the real scale of the social consequences for men and women (ROCHA, 2000).

There is no single, global strategy that is valid for the whole of society and applies uniformly to all manifestations of sex: the idea, for example, that we have often tried, by different means, to reduce all sex to its reproductive function, to its adult form, does not in the least explain the multiple objectives pursued, the countless means put into action in sexual policies concerning the two sexes, different ages and social classes (FOUCAULT, 2014, p. 112).112).

Practices related to caring for the sick have been around for as long as humans have existed, and it is impossible to pinpoint a specific date for their origins. It is known that these practices were carried out by amateurs, without any training or sufficient information to care for or even medicate the sick. As man entered society, work became increasingly central to his survival and coexistence (NOGUEIRA, 2011).

The development and use of knowledge is essential for the constant improvement not only of patient care but also of health itself, in order to base nursing actions and decisions on evidence that indicates that they are appropriate, bringing positive results for all (POLIT, 2004).

The current transformations in the world of work have had direct consequences on the lives and health of workers, incisively and, for the most part, negatively, since the increased pace of work means that they consume physical and psychological energy, leading them to develop stress in their personal and professional lives (MARTINS, 2014).

And when we look at the distribution of men and women in employment, but also in training careers, the "technical" criterion appears to be extremely discriminatory (MARUANI, HIRATA, 2003).

For a better understanding, Melo (1986) shows that understanding the organization of work in nursing is intrinsically related to questions of the distribution of functions and tasks, and consequently to the division of labour.

Lobo (1991) mentions that the sexuality of jobs goes through a complex cultural mechanism that defines "women's courses" and "men's courses", but much more than that, through different hierarchical and quality relations between the sexes, representations of responsibility and suitability, which in turn refer to power relations based on the technical knowledge inherent in the job.

Fangyi (2015) adds that studying the individual occupation of nursing professionals provides a contribution to a range of other different occupational groups, where we can associate work and shift routines with different occupational diseases.

Nursing work is first and foremost a way of being in the midst of diffuse emotions. Emotions that are received from those who are being cared for, as well as from the entire team that is involved in providing care around the clock. And much of the care provided by the team is sometimes based on the foundation of the patient's suffering, as well as the internal relationships of each nurse with that patient

(SANTOS, 2002).

As nursing professionals are committed to caring for others and improving their quality of life, it is of fundamental importance that they have good living and working conditions (FONTANA, 2015).

1.5 NIGHT WORK

It is in this context that the activity of the nursing team and night work is inserted, and as much as the relationship between health and quality of life is obvious, it is pertinent and relevant to study the subject of the daily lives of many professionals, health or not.

According to data from the Ministry of Labor, it is estimated that in Brazil there are around 15 million night workers, and according to WHO surveys, more than 20% of the populations of developed and developing countries work in the early hours of the morning. And although night work is harmful to workers' health, it's important to note that we have legislation that provides for the right of all professionals to receive compensation, both in terms of hours and wages, for their night work.

Parafo and Martino (2004) point out that the low salaries of the nursing staff contribute directly to the promotion of double shifts in order to increase income and contribute to a better family situation. As a result of this physical and psychological strain, it would not be difficult to find professionals on the verge of the symptoms inherent in organizational stress (RODRIGUES, 2015).

Silva (2011) comments on the social roles of each individual and their personal consequences, because due to the basic condition of being human, nursing professionals need to manipulate two parallel paths that intersect at all times in the workplace. On the one hand, there is family and social life, and on the other, life inside hospitals and health centers, which is often difficult to control.

Since hospital work has a continuity factor, i.e. the presence of healthcare workers is required on a permanent basis, the same also happens at night. The point is that workers exposed to abnormal working hours can suffer consequences such as reduced cognitive functions due to partial or total sleep deprivation (HORN; COTANDA, 2011).

In today's contemporary society, night work is necessary and important, thus requiring demand throughout the day in critical services such as public security, politics, firefighting, health, transportation, communication, electricity, water and fuel, among others (CHERE, 2016).

And when we talk about work, specifically the adaptation to working in different shifts as one of the forms of temporal organization of work through shifts and night work, where the same activity must be performed at different times of the day and night by several other employees on a similar journey (FILHO, 2004).

Gender has a strong influence on tolerance to shift work, acting more through social than biological means. Among those who work at night, important changes need to be made, such as reorganizing their routine to accommodate sleep and the other activities that make up their lives during the day, which is more complex for women, due to the role traditionally attributed to them in terms of the home and family. It is worth mentioning that the unequal division of domestic work between men and women is not always reflected in different degrees of tolerance to shift work (FISCHER, 2003).

Hospital work is divided into shifts, and care must be provided 24 hours a day, 7 days a week without any interruption. This means that hospitals have to be on alert regardless of commemorative dates, holidays or weekends, forcing employees to take turns in order to maintain a "normal" social life (PARAFO; MARTINO, 2004).

> Life on Earth depends on the presence of the sun and due to the rotation of our planet around its own axis, or around the sun, all organisms on the Earth's surface are subjected to different intensities of light throughout the 24 hours and seasons of the year. Thus, the alternation of light and dark, atmospheric conditions, ambient temperature and the seasons of the year play an important role in regulating daily (circadian or nicteremal), weekly (circassertive), seasonal (seasonal) and annual (circannual) physiological rhythms. And during the evolution of living beings, from the simplest forms of prokaryotes, organisms, dependent on sunlight, adapted their way of life, adjusting their period of activity to obtain greater survival, and began to organize their activities in 24-hour cycles determined by the rising and setting of the sun (JANSEN, 2007, p.71).

Cheres (2016) reports that night work has existed since the dawn of human history, when prehistoric man needed to meet the survival needs of his family group when he went out to hunt at night.

And with the invention of fire, around 7000 B.C., humans were better able to work at night, outside their shelters, so that they could carry out vigilante activities, such as guarding fields and shepherding their flocks.

Shift work is one of the major deteriorators in the quality of life of various professional categories, especially considering that many health workers end up having two jobs in order to survive in a way that is considered dignified (HORN; COTANDA, 2011).

Rotenberg (2003) mentions that day and night working hours had already been established several centuries ago, especially in industrial, extractive and health service activities. For this reason, the spread of the double working day is not an extinct condition in the nursing team. Many professionals need this routine because of financial difficulties.

Night work is a necessary part of everyday life, but it entails a number of risks to workers' health, both biologically and psychologically, and among other emotional problems, making them more prone to stress, anxiety attacks and emotional fatigue. This is due to the inversion of the biological clock, which not only causes harmful consequences for workers' health but also disrupts family relationships (CHERES, 2016).

Horn and Contada (2011) confirm that working at night also causes physiological disorders related to sleep disturbances, which are aggravated by the fact that workers are unable to rest properly after planting due to the noise and brightness of the domestic environment, as well as appetite disturbances and digestive problems, since daytime sleep does not have the same restorative effects as nighttime sleep.

In addition, the night shift is harmful to sleep and health, as well as to family life, which is intensified when hospital workers who work at night have other professional activities during the day.

Abreu (2012) states that for night workers, sleep time is often seen as insufficient, especially at weekends and on days off, as there is an attempt to compensate for those who don't sleep during the day so that they can take advantage of their family commitments.

In other words, the worker is already tired from the day's work and is still working at night. The change in the biological clock exposes the worker to a greater number of risks than daytime work, requiring another organization of daily life, among other aspects, and demanding another formulation of life, very different from the possible and appropriate formulations for activities carried out in other economic segments (HORN; COTANDA, 2011).

Night work is an activity that requires the employee to perform services or activities at night for the employer, who will have a percentage of 20% added to their salary for each hour worked. Our legislation defines night work as that performed between 10 p.m. one day and 5 a.m. the next (CHERES, 2016).

So, when we talk about the legal aspect of regulating night work, it is necessary to mention that the Federal Constitution (CF) in its article 7, item IX, establishes that workers' rights are to be paid more for night work than for day work. Article 73 of the Consolidation of Labor Laws (CLT) states:

> Art. 73: Except in the case of weekly or fortnightly shifts, night work shall be paid more than day work and, for this purpose, its remuneration shall be increased by at least 20% (twenty percent) over the daytime hour. (Editing given by Decree-Law no. 9.666, of 1946)
>
> § Paragraph 1. The hour of night work shall be computed as 52 minutes and 30 seconds. (Editing given by Decree-Law no. 9.666, of 1946)
>
> § Paragraph 2. For the purposes of this article, work performed between 10 p.m. on one day and 5 a.m. on the following day is considered night work.
>
> § Paragraph 3 - The increase referred to in this article, in the case of companies which do not, due to the nature of their activities, regularly work at night, shall be made taking into account the amounts paid for daytime work of a similar nature. In the case of companies whose night work is due to the nature of their activities, the increase will be calculated on the general minimum wage in force in the region, and will not be due when it exceeds this limit, already increased by the percentage. (Editing given by Decree-Law no. 9.666, of 1946)
>
> § Paragraph 4. In the case of mixed working hours, i.e. those covering both day and night periods, the provisions of this article and its paragraphs shall apply to night work hours. (Editing by Decree-Law No. 9.666, of 1946)
>
> § Paragraph 5. The provisions of this chapter shall apply to extensions of night work. (Included by Decree-Law No. 9.666, of 1946) (BRASIL, 2016).

And from the perspective of nursing, Braga (2015) states that nurses and the nursing team, unable to work out these favorable conditions, do not benefit from the work to master their suffering and transform it into creativity, causing wear and tear on the job.

It can be said that working at night can be considered an additional risk factor for the development of health problems and an increase in the number of typical accidents, since sleep deprivation caused by difficulty in resting during the day can significantly reduce workers' alertness levels and accentuate symptoms of fatigue (HORN; COTANDA, 2011).

Night work is extremely important nowadays, due to its generous application and being for technical, social and economic reasons, but it is worth noting that this temporal organization of work can generate various health risks for those who work during this period, as several studies have shown that various disorders, diseases or problems are more likely to be caused to workers who perform night activities (CHERES, 2016).

If, on the one hand, shift work has many positive points for the growing demands of a society that is on the move 24 hours a day, on the other hand, for shift workers it means "paying a high price", as it requires extra attention and produces tension, fatigue and sleep disorders.

This happens despite the adoption of measures to reduce the impact on health and safety at work, such as reducing the number of hours and adopting shift rotas that favor the body's recovery.

Thus, the benefits offered to those who work at night, such as additional night pay, overtime and more free time during the day, do not compensate for the immediate and long-term effects on their health of the wear and tear of working in conditions that subvert the biological clock (JANSEN, 2007).

Based on these premises, we intend to try to identify the impacts that night work has on the quality of life of male nursing professionals, believing that we can contribute to a better assessment of workers' issues by pointing out some possible realities that could be changed.

It is up to health professionals "to give visibility to these processes, to unveil their impacts and damage and to build so that the rights already won are guaranteed and expanded" (PIGNATI, et al., 2013, p.379).

According to a study on night work and its repercussions on the health of nurses, the shift requires the worker to be aware of their physical limits in order to carry out the activity and not interfere with the disease process, much less compromise the quality of care provided. Furthermore, it is necessary to adopt measures to reduce the impact on health in order to improve the safety of those who work at night (SILVA et al., 2011).

In another study, Silva et al (2014) reflected that these workers experience a series of situations that compromise their daytime rest, such as micro-awakenings, the numerous sounds in the environment and sunlight. As a result, alarming figures show that night workers live less than those who work during the day, and that those who work at night lose five years of life for every 15 years worked.

Fangy (2015) mentions that there is recognition of the many links between shift work and health problems, and the role that circadian rhythm plays in vascular health and tumor prevention is clear, as this relationship is potentially harmful between night shift work and health.

And even though shift work involves unavoidable problems, as it goes against biological principles and social coexistence, understanding the issues surrounding this activity and the adverse effects of working hours.

However, it is necessary not only to cite solutions to these problems, but to study the reality of many professionals and propose recommendations for minimizing workers' difficulties in terms of health and psychosocial well-being, in order to enable them to cope with their work shift while trying to reduce its consequences on their lives.

2 METHODOLOGICAL PATH

2.1 TYPE OF RESEARCH

This is a descriptive, cross-sectional study with a quantitative approach. When combined, the use of quantitative techniques for both data collection and analysis allows more significant conclusions to be drawn from the data collected, which enables better strategic planning for the adoption of conduct and forms of action in different contexts (FREITAS; MOSCAROLA, 2002).

The concern with knowledge of reality is a constant in human life, since research is a form of investigation that aims to find answers to society's questions through scientific procedures (BEUREN, 2004).

Lakatos (2010) states that it is from the relationship that man has with the world, in his constant questioning and inquiry, in whatever field, that important elements arise, such as awareness and knowledge of the reality of the experiences of his social group. However, science uses its own method, the scientific method, which is a fundamental element of the process of knowledge carried out by science to differentiate it not only from common sense, but also from other forms of expression of human subjectivity (SEVERINO, 2007).

Thus, the act of research is defined by Vieira (2015) as being a systematic procedure of investigation carried out to review or expand existing knowledge, discovering new facts, discussing new ways of thinking, rectifying old conclusions and developing new technologies.

In this context, nursing research is essential for the nursing team to understand the various dimensions present in their profession, as it allows them to describe the characteristics of a particular nursing situation about which little is known, in an attempt to explain phenomena that must be considered in order to determine the probable results of certain common decisions in their professional activity (POLIT, 2004).

There is no doubt that research, at the same time as producing knowledge, has triggered great progress in nursing and that without it the countless social, scientific, intellectual, technical and professional achievements of the nursing team would not have been possible (OGUISSO, 2007).

Investigations that produce "snapshots" of the health situation of a population or community, based on the individual assessment of the health status of each member of the group, thus producing global health indicators for the group investigated, are called sectional or cross-sectional studies (SILVA, ROUQUAYROL, 2014).

Therefore, cross-sectional studies require a precise and concise definition of the object of study and the simpler the objective, the easier it will be to carry out the study and with fewer possibilities for errors (HADDAD, 2004).

However, Polit (2004) points out that the main concern of quantitative research in its methodology is to provide accurate, impartial and interpretable answers to the research question through good methodological design, thereby providing valid and replicable results.

Quantitative research aims to count, order and measure in order to establish the frequency and distribution of phenomena, in order to look for patterns of relationships between variables, test hypotheses and establish confidence intervals for error parameters for estimates. Quantitative researchers therefore look for numerical data that can be analyzed (VIEIRA, 2015).

2.2 FIELD OF RESEARCH

The setting chosen was the Hospital de Clinicas da Universidade Federal de Uberlândia- HC/UFU, located in the state of Minas Gerais. It is a general public teaching hospital with 525 beds, offering a wide range of medium and high complexity health services to users of the Unified Health System (SUS), and is a reference point for the wider Northern Triangle region with an estimated population of 1,200,000 inhabitants.

2.3 RESEARCH SUBJECTS

The study population consisted of 72 male nursing staff (nurses, technicians and nursing assistants) working at the HC/UFU during the night, with a 12/36 working week. All agreed to answer the questionnaire. As for the losses, one professional refused on the grounds that he was embarrassed and had previous experience in other research where the researcher didn't like his answers.

Currently, the Nursing Directorate has more than 1214 professionals, including 189 nurses, 963 technicians and nursing assistants. Of these, 74 professionals are male and work at night, so as one refused and the other was the researcher, the study population was 72 participants, and the questionnaire was applied to 100% of the population.

On the other hand, Lakatos (2010) states that it is not always possible to carry out research with all the individuals in the group or community you wish to study, due to a lack of resources or time constraints.

When talking about determining sample size, Lobiondo-Wood (2001) states that there is no single rule that can be applied when determining sample size, since many factors inherent to the study are taken into account when arriving at an estimate.

According to Haddad (2004), in cross-sectional studies, by defining the sample, we can present some advantages such as a reduced cost, because it is not carried out on a smaller number of individuals; a shorter time for its execution, in addition to allowing a greater number of data to be collected, thus reducing the possibility of errors during the development of the study.

It is very important to carefully define the inclusion and exclusion criteria, because they establish the population to which the results will be generalized (VIEIRA, 2015).

Some inclusion and exclusion criteria were established for the study, which included male nursing professionals with the position of nurse, technician and nursing assistants, who work at night on a 12/36 hour shift, in the care units of the Hospital de Clinicas de Uberlândia.

On the other hand, the following nursing professionals were excluded: females; those working day shifts: afternoon and/or morning; those working night shifts as on-call staff and those who did not agree to the research and did not sign the Informed Consent Form (Appendix A).

2.4 DATA COLLECTION

The selection of the methodological instrument is one of the most important phases of a study and is directly related to the problem to be studied, and its choice will depend on various factors and elements related to the investigation (LAKATOS, 2010).

The questionnaires were applied on the basis of pre-calculated sampling in accordance with the laws of statistical probability, so that the possibilities of error are minimal, and the results of the sample are certainly extended to the universe of subjects involved in the study (ALVES; SANTOS, 2014).

For Severino (2007), a questionnaire is a set of systematically articulated questions designed to elicit written information from research subjects, with a view to ascertaining their opinion on the issues under study". Lakatos (2010) defines a questionnaire as a data collection instrument consisting of an ordered series of questions to be answered in writing.

As for the advantages of the instrument, Alves and Santos (2014) list as its main advantages the possibility of being carried out simultaneously in several places and with several informants; it allows for comparisons; anonymity is ensured more easily and understood by the respondent, as they know that there will be several others answering the questions on the questionnaire, and contact with the researcher is more objective; tabulation and analysis of the data is faster and more accurate, including through the use of statistical programs such as the Statistical Package for Social Sciences (SPSS).

To assess various factors, individual questionnaires can be used with the workers and observations can also be made at the workstations, as this is a method that makes it possible to survey the list of difficulties perceived at work, providing a more reliable basis for any intervention or assessment aimed at eliminating certain non-conformities inherent in the professional activity (ROCHA, 2012).

In the quantitative approach to assessing quality of life, the Word Health Quality of Life (WHOQOL-breve) instrument was used, an abbreviated instrument for assessing quality of life (Appendix-B), developed by the World Health Organization and validated and adapted for Brazil.

Oguisso (2007) explains that the World Health Organization (WHO) is a governmental entity linked to the United Nations (UN) and follows the same basic principles of harmonious relations and security for all peoples.

The WHOQOL-bref or abbreviated WHOQOL is an alternative generic quality of life measurement instrument that is short, applicable to any population, can be answered regardless of level of education and allows the researcher to include other measures of interest in addition to quality of life (FLECK, 2008).

Variables such as age (in years), marital status, job title and length of service (in years) were added at the beginning of the questionnaire. A minimum of 8 and a maximum of 15 minutes was estimated for the questionnaire.

This instrument contains twenty-six questions that assess five domains, using a response scale. The Likert scale is used, as it measures attitudes and behaviors using response options that vary from one extreme to another. In other words, for each question, the examiner asks you to circle the number that best answers it, with 5 alternatives such as: 1- very bad, 2- bad, 3- neither bad nor good, 4- good, 5- very good. Unlike a simple "yes or no" question, a Likert scale makes it possible to discover more specific levels of opinion.

Below is a description of each domain and the facets of each domain: PHYSICAL - pain, energy, sleep, mobility, activities of daily living, dependence on medication/treatment, ability to work; PSYCHOLOGICAL - positive/negative feelings, thoughts, self-esteem, body image, spirituality; SOCIAL RELATIONSHIPS - personal relationships, social support and sexual activity; ENVIRONMENT - physical safety, home environment, financial resources, health and social care, opportunities to acquire information and skills, recreation/leisure, physical environment and transportation; GENERAL - overall quality of life and general health perceptions. The score is obtained by adding up the options that the respondent ticks (FLECK, 2008).

Thus, we can understand a domain as a set of themes that a variable can take, and a facet as a smaller part, in other words, the first would be a general theme or subject and the second as a sub-theme, both directly related to QoL. In the case of the facets we have to measure all the scores for each item, and these range from 4 to 20, with higher scores denoting higher quality of life, except for the reverse score facets, such as pain and discomfort, negative feelings and dependence on medication.

To measure quality of life, we have a scale of 0 to 100, and the closer you are to this average, the better quality of life you have. It is very difficult to correlate other values as parameters, because the study population is very specific and there are few studies using the same methodology.

The data was collected by the researchers in charge and took place in January 2016, during the night shift and during working hours. The participation of the professionals was voluntary and anonymous, and the invitation took place during their shift and dinner times. At the time, the objectives, methodologies and ethical aspects of the research were explained. Those who wished to take part answered the questionnaire in the sector itself, after signing the Informed Consent Form (Appendix A), which contained detailed information about the study, the freedom to withdraw from the study at any time, a guarantee of anonymity and confirmation that there would be no harm or complications for the participants.

2.5 DATA ANALYSIS PROCEDURES

The sample data was tabulated in electronic spreadsheets and summarized using descriptive statistics, and presented in tables and figures as means ± standard deviation (quantitative data), while categorical variables will be expressed as absolute or relative frequencies. Statistical analysis will be carried out using the Statistical Package for the Social Science (SPSS), version 22.0.

Obtaining precise answers in the search for information results from exhaustive work that requires knowledge and skills in research techniques (MINEO, 2005). Defining variables is an important and necessary task in order to direct data analysis. Vieira (2015) states that a variable is any characteristic or attribute that can have different values when different individuals are observed and data is a value assumed by the variable when an individual is examined.

The quantitative variables were described using the mean, median, maximum and minimum standard deviation. In addition, the Shapiro-Wilk normality test was applied. As the variables did not follow a normal distribution, the Kruskall-Wallis test was applied. The qualitative variables were described (frequency and percentage) using frequency tables. Associations between quantitative variables were measured using Spearman's correlation coefficient (ZAR, 1999). All tests were carried out using SPSS software (v.20) and considering a significance level of 5% ($p < 0.05$).

The Shapiro-Wilk test is used to check whether the data follow a normal distribution, and is more suitable for small samples; the Kruskall-Wallis test is a statistical procedure that aims to compare three or more independent samples of the same or unequal size whose scores are measured at ordinal levels; the Spearman coefficient is a test that involves calculating the statistical value by means of procedures and formulas to define averages and variations between the relationships of the given variables (FONTELLES, 2012).

2.6 ETHICAL ASPECTS

Research Ethics Committees (RECs) are councils that review research projects to assess whether certain ethical standards have been met in relation to protecting the rights of human beings (LOBIONDO-WOOD, 2001).

Even so, Vieira (2015) informs us that CEP's are multidisciplinary, as they are made up of professionals from different areas, representatives of the community and representatives of users of the institution's health system, so in Brazil, no researcher can start a study on human beings without proper approval from a CEP.

In all research work on human beings, the individual must be informed of the objectives, methods, expected advantages and risks inherent in the study, as well as the inconveniences it may entail. However, the individual can abstain from taking part in the study and is free to withdraw their consent at any time (HADDAD, 2004).

The study was submitted to the Research Ethics Committee of the Federal University of Uberlândia-MG for analysis and an informed consent form (APPENDIX-A) was obtained from all respondents in accordance with Resolution 466/12 of the National Health Council. The study received a favorable opinion from the Certificate of Submission for Ethical Appraisal (CAAE) under no. 50235515.9.0000.5152 on December 17, 2015.

3 RESULTS AND DISCUSSION

Every year, nursing has been increasingly sought after by men who are interested in the practice of care. And yet, with all the changes in habits and in the social, political and economic conjunctures, it is still seen that the job market and also in scientific studies there is little action and production on the gender issue, specifically in the nursing profession.

Believing in the importance of this approach to nursing workers who work at night and the impact on their quality of life, we initially looked at some figures to justify the study.

Figure 2: Explanation of the study context.

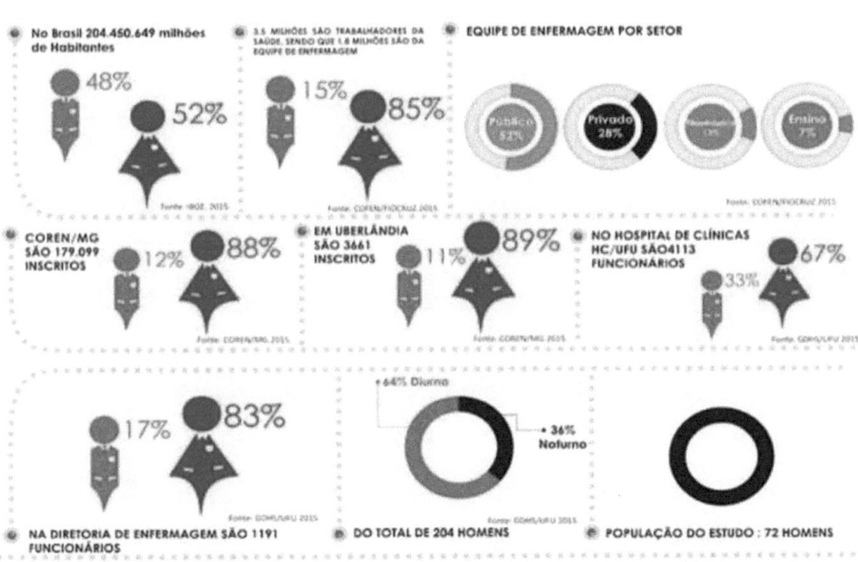

Source: Researchers' database (2016).

It is important to mention that the findings were based on figures from the Brazilian Institute of Statistics and Geography (IBGE) and in the specific case of secondary data from the Hospital de Clinicas de Uberlândia (HC/UFU), from the Human Resources and Development Management sector (GDHS/UFU), the Transparency Portal and also from the "Profile of Nursing in Brazil" survey

- a survey carried out in partnership between the Osvaldo Cruz Foundation (FIOCRUZ) and the Federal Nursing Council (COFEN).

Figure 2 presents a numerical survey of the issue of gender and nursing, in an attempt to contextualize it in a chronological and contextual way, from the macro issue to the importance of the sample in this study.

According to estimates by the IBGE (2015), Brazil has more than 204 million inhabitants, 48% of whom are male. Of the total number of inhabitants, more than 3.5 million are health workers, of whom more than 1.8 million are nursing staff.

The numbers justify the large presence of the profession and its team within health establishments, showing its importance, and it is most present in the public health sector (52%), followed by the private (28%), philanthropic (13%) and teaching (7%) sectors (COFEN/FIOCRUZ, 2015).

In addition, the number of professionals registered with the Regional Nursing Council in Minas Gerais (COREN/MG) in 2015 was over 179,000, and the number of men was 12%; those registered with the section in Uberlândia/MG, the site of the study, were over 3,600 professionals, with only 11% men; and in the sector of the study, which was a large hospital, there were more than 4,100 employees, 33% of whom were men, and more than 1,91 employees working in the Nursing Department, 17% of whom were men.

And by restricting this universe to 204 men, after surveying them, we found that 64% of them work during the day and 36% at night (leaving 72 men, who make up 100% of the study population) (GDHS, 2015).

Thus, all 72 nursing professionals answered the questionnaire, with the highest number of nursing technicians (41 - 56.9%), followed by nursing assistants (18 - 25%) and nurses (13 - 18.1%). In a comparison with the national study, these figures corroborate the COFEN/FIOCRUZ survey (2013), in which we can state that the majority of the nursing team is made up of 77% nursing technicians and assistants, followed by 23% nurses in their workforce.

Table 1: Description of the variables: marital status, employment relationship, help with filling in and position (N=72).

Variables		n	%
CIVIL STATUS	married	42	58,3
	divorced	3	4,2
	separate	1	1,4
	single	26	36,1
ViNCULO	FAEPU	22	30,6
	UFU	50	69,4
GET HELP	No	72	100,0
ROLE	Aux Enf	18	25,0
	Nurse	13	18,1
	Tec Enf	41	56,9

Source: Prepared by the researchers, study data, 2016.

Table 1 shows the variables added to the study and the prevalence of married marital status, 42 (58.3%), 26 (36.1%) were single, followed by 3 (4.2%) divorced and 1 (1.4%) separated. It can be seen that the majority are married and the minority are separated or divorced. Data from a European study states that night workers live less and divorce more, and may be three times more likely to divorce and more than 40% more likely to become ill (LINDA et al., 2014).

Current data shows that the nursing profession is in full rejuvenation, with ¼ of its contingent being up to 30 years old, making it clear that they are mostly starting out in the job market and their professional lives (MACHADO et al., 2016).

In terms of employment, 69.4% were UFU employees working under the Single Juridical Regime (RJU) and 30.6% were employees of the Foundation for Support and Research (FAEPU) working under the Consolidation of Labor

Laws (CLT). Machado et al. (2016) states that nursing work today is concentrated within hospitals, and more than 1 million of them work in the three spheres of government, making the public sector the largest employer in the category, followed by the private, philanthropic and teaching sectors, as shown in figure 2.

One of the questions on the questionnaire asked whether help was needed to fill it in. The data showed that 100% did not need any help; the average time taken was 7.18 minutes to complete the questionnaire, with 4 minutes being the shortest and 20 minutes the longest. It is worth mentioning that the methodology of the study estimated an average time of 7 to 15 minutes to answer, thus showing the validity of the instrument, since it is self-administered and help could interfere with the answers when filling it in.

Fleck (2008) points out that the questionnaire is self-answering, and that the interviewer should not influence or discuss the choice of answers, much less avoid giving synonyms to the words in the questions in order to avoid influencing the individual's judgment.

The description of the categorical variables (marital status, employment relationship, help with filling in the questionnaire and job title) is shown in Table 1. The description of the quantitative variables (age, length of service and time taken to complete the questionnaire) is shown in Table 2.

Table 2. Description of the variables: age, length of service and time spent filling in the questionnaire.

	Media	Median	Standard deviation	Minimum	Maximum	Normality
AGE (years)	40,32	38,50	10,138	19	66	0,004
LENGTH OF SERVICE	16,39	14,00	10,822	1	40	0,011
FILLING TIME (in minutes)	7,18	5,00	3,396	4	20	0,001

Source: Prepared by the researchers, database obtained from WHOQOL-brev (2016).

The average age was 40.32 years, with the lowest being 19 years and the highest 66 years; the average length of service in the institution was 16.39 years, making it clear that the majority of the team has a great deal of professional experience. On the other hand, the shortest time was 1 year and the longest was 40 years of service; with regard to filling time, the average was 7.18 minutes, with a minimum of 4 minutes and a maximum of 20 minutes.

We can say that the predominant types of contract or employment relationship among the nursing team are the federal public sector, governed by the RJU, with over a million professionals, followed by the CLT. In relation to average age and length of service, we can correlate the data with their employment contracts, as the majority have been civil servants for longer in the same activity and institution.

Table 3 shows the normality of the questionnaire domains (DOMI- Physical, DOM2- Psychological, DOM3- Social Relations, DOM4- Environment, DOM5- Self-assessment of QoL, GENERAL) using the Shapiro-Wilk test and none of these variables follow a normal probability distribution ($p < 0.05$).

Table 3. Correlation between the variables age, length of service and time spent completing the questionnaire *versus the* questionnaire domains.

		DOMI	DOM2	DOM3	DOM4	DOM5	GENERAL
AGE	Correlation	0,144	0,062	0,025	-0,084	0,199	0,032
	p value	0,227	0,607	0,837	0,481	0,093	0,788
TIME OF	Correlation	0,107	0,058	-0,015	0,007	0,136	0,044
SERVICE	p value	0,369	0,629	0,901	0,953	0,256	0,716
TIME OF	Correlation	0,041	0,009	-0,039	-0,132	-0,012	-0,033
FILL IN	p value	0,730	0,943	0,745	0,269	0,920	0,780

Source: Prepared by the researchers, database obtained from WHOQOL-brev, 2016.

Thus, all the tests used were non-parametric. As a result, when correlating the variables age, length of service and time spent filling out the questionnaire with each domain, there were no significant changes, leaving the same average between them.

The categorical variables, grouped with the results and in certain questions (job title, position) showed no significant differences or changes.

Table 4 shows the comparisons of the marital status of nursing professionals in relation to the domains of the questionnaire. It can be seen that there is no significant difference ($p > 0.05$) between the marital status of the professionals in relation to each domain of the questionnaire, so marital status does not interfere with the domains.

In other words, the comparison of marital status in relation to the domains shows that regardless of marital status, the domains of social relationships and self-assessment of quality of life prevailed. It is worth noting that in all the scores analyzed, married people had a higher index than single people and divorced/separated people. It can be concluded that the quality of life of married people is higher, although there are minimal differences, and these are representative and important.

Another relevant fact to highlight is that the comparisons of the scores shown in the following tables show that regardless of the variable in relation to the tabulated domains, they did not show a difference that altered the general scope in terms of measuring the quality of life of the study group. The debate thus becomes clearer with the analysis of the facets of each domain.

Table 4. Comparison of marital status in relation to the questionnaire domains

		n	Media	Median	Standard deviation	Minimum	Maximum
DOM1 (Physicist)	Married	42	14,89796	15,42857	2,55361	9,14286	18,85714
	Divorced/ Separated	4	13,71429	13,14286	3,02372	10,85714	17,71429
	Single	26	13,89011	14,28571	3,04853	8,00000	18,85714
	p value			0,293			

DOM2 (Psychological)	Married	42	15,28571	15,33333	2,52636	8,66667	19,33333
	Divorced/ Separated	4	13,66667	15,00000	3,37749	8,66667	16,00000
	Single	26	14,23077	14,66667	2,59190	8,00000	18,00000
	p value			0,139			
DOM3 (Relations Social)	Married	42	15,55556	16,00000	3,18079	6,66667	20,00000
	Divorced/ Separated	4	15,33333	15,33333	1,72133	13,33333	17,33333
	Single	26	14,66667	15,33333	3,20000	8,00000	20,00000
	p value			0,467			
DOM4 (Middle Environment)	Married	42	13,55952	13,75000	2,66916	8,00000	19,00000
	Divorced/ Separated	4	13,37500	12,75000	2,17466	11,50000	16,50000
	Single	p26	12,57692	12,25000	2,40704	7,50000	18,00000
	value			0,281			
DOM5 (Self-assessment of QoL)	Married	42	13,23810	14,00000	4,11902	6,00000	20,00000
	Divorced/ Separated	4	12,50000	11,00000	3,78594	10,00000	18,00000
	Single	26	12,92308	12,00000	3,00564	8,00000	18,00000
	p value			0,850			
GENERAL	Married	42	14,52381	14,84615	2,27888	8,30769	18,46154
	Divorced/ Separated	4	13,69231	13,61538	2,51544	10,76923	16,76923
	Single	26	13,57988	14,00000	2,16286	8,15385	18,30769
	p value			0,145			

Source: Prepared by the researchers, database obtained from WHOQOL-brev, 2016

Table 5 shows the comparisons of the nursing professionals' jobs in relation to the questionnaire's domains. It can be seen that there is no significant difference (p > 0.05) between the professionals' positions in relation to each domain of the questionnaire, so the position does not interfere with the domains.

Table 5. Comparison of position in relation to questionnaire domains

		n	Media	Median	Standard deviation	Minimum	Maximum
DOM1 (Physicist)	Aux Enf	18	14,47619	14,85714	2,84704	9,14286	18,28571
	Nurse	13	14,54945	14,28571	2,91013	10,28571	18,85714
	Tec Enf	41	14,43902	14,85714	2,76723	8,00000	18,85714
	p value			0,994			
DOM2 (Psychological)	Aux Enf	18	14,66667	14,66667	2,18132	10,00000	18,00000
	Nurse	13	14,61538	15,33333	2,68689	8,66667	18,00000
	Tec Enf	41	14,94309	15,33333	2,82046	8,00000	19,33333
	p value			0,587			
DOM3 (Relations Social)	Aux Enf	18	14,88889	15,33333	3,80574	8,00000	20,00000
	Nurse	13	15,17949	16,00000	2,75081	10,66667	20,00000
	Tec Enf	41	15,38211	16,00000	2,96794	6,66667	20,00000
	p value			0,812			
DOM4 (Middle Environment)	Aux Enf	18	13,50000	13,25000	2,54951	9,50000	18,00000
	Nurse	13	13,84615	13,50000	2,15430	10,00000	18,00000
	Tec Enf	41	12,85366	12,50000	2,68618	7,50000	19,00000
	p value			0,369			
DOM5 (Self-evaluation of QL)	Aux Enf	18	13,22222	14,00000	3,63893	6,00000	18,00000
	Nurse	13	12,76923	12,00000	3,70031	8,00000	18,00000

	Tec Enf	41	13,12195	14,00000	3,79602	6,00000	20,00000
	p value			0,912			
GENERAL	Aux Enf	18	14,17094	14,00000	2,30672	10,15385	18,00000
	Nurse	13	14,28402	14,46154	2,32459	10,76923	18,30769
	Tec Enf	41	14,07505	14,61538	2,28168	8,15385	18,46154
	p value			0,976			

Source: Prepared by the researchers, database obtained from WHOQOL-brev, 2016.

Table 6 shows the comparisons of nursing professionals' relationships in relation to the questionnaire's domains. It can be seen that there is no significant difference ($p > 0.05$) between the professionals' relationships in relation to each domain of the questionnaire, so the relationship does not interfere with the domains.

Table 6. Comparison of bonding in relation to the questionnaire domains

		n	Media	Median	Standard deviation	Minimum	Maximum
DOM1 (Physicist)	FAEPU	22	14,23377	14,28571	3,05904	8,00000	18,85714
	UFU	50	14,57143	14,85714	2,66340	8,57143	18,85714
	p value			0,650			
DOM2 (Psychological)	FAEPU	22	14,51515	15,00000	2,71334	8,00000	18,00000
	UFU	50	14,94667	15,33333	2,59457	8,00000	19,33333
	p value			0,494			
DOM3 (Social Relations)	FAEPU	22	15,09091	16,00000	2,51594	10,66667	20,00000
	UFU	50	15,28000	16,00000	3,37750	6,66667	20,00000
	p value			0,704			
DOM4 (Environment)	FAEPU	22	13,13636	13,25000	2,34105	9,00000	18,00000
	UFU	50	13,22000	13,00000	2,67864	7,50000	19,00000
	p value			0,971			
DOM5 (Self-evaluation of							

QL)	FAEPU	22	12,63636	12,00000	3,82405	6,00000	18,00000
	UFU	50	13,28000	14,00000	3,65357	6,00000	20,00000
	p value			0,520			
GENERAL	FAEPU	22	13,93706	14,53846	2,18381	10,30769	18,30769
	UFU	50	14,22462	14,46154	2,31495	8,15385	18,46154
	p value			0,590			

Source: Prepared by the researchers, database obtained from WHOQOL-brev, 2016.

Table 7 shows the Spearman correlation coefficients between the quantitative variables (age, length of service and time spent completing the questionnaire) *and* the questionnaire domains. It can be seen that there is no significant correlation, so these variables do not correlate directly with the questionnaire domains.

With the descriptive statistical evaluation of the data in relation to the instrument, the average for each domain shows that the social relations domain stood out, followed by the psychological and physical domains, with the lowest average for the environment and self-assessment of quality of life domains. We can say that these figures show that the data relating to the consolidated scores allows them to be correlated with the characteristics of the study population.

Even though it is used as a base, the average for an analysis of the scores shows that the standard deviation changed little and that only two domains had a maximum value of 20, social relations and self-assessment, a number that should be described as a percentage, since the sum of them will be 100%.

Table 7. Descriptive statistics (mean, standard deviation, coefficient of variation, maximum, minimum and range) of the quality of life scores of the team of nursing professionals.

DOMAIN	AVERAGE	STANDARD DEVIATION	COEFFICIENT VARIATION	MINIMUM VALUE	MAXIMUM VALUE	AMPLITUDE
Physical	14,47	2,77	19,16	8,00	18,86	10,86
Psychological	14,81	2,62	17,68	8,00	19,33	11,33
Relationships						

Social	15,22	3,12	20,52	6,67	20,00	13,33
Medium						
Environment	13,19	2,56	19,43	7,50	19,00	11,50
Auto evaluation of QL	13,08	3,69	28,21	6,00	20,00	14,00
TOTAL	14,14	2,26	16,02	8,15	18,46	10,31

Source: Prepared by the researchers, database obtained from WHOQOL-brev, 2016.

The domains and their facets show that the population studied reveals details that often go unnoticed by managers and sectors, as in the case of Human Resources and the Workers' Health Sector. In terms of numbers, the nursing team in the health sectors, especially in the care sector, has a large contingent of people, a minority of whom are men.

In order to measure and evaluate the aspects of this group, it is necessary to correlate them with other issues inherent to professional activity, since the particularities and specificities have many direct effects on the quality of life of these professionals. In Table 2 and Table 3, we give an overview of how and where the potential, conflicts and difficulties of this universe of analysis originate.

Graph 1 shows a general consolidation of the results found in each domain. In other words, in a representation of the domains and their respective values, social relations, psychological, physical, general and environment prevailed in chronological order. Graph 2 shows the grouping of the facets in the WHOQOL-Abbreviated questionnaire according to the values obtained in the survey. The yellow colors mean the lowest values, and the facets marked with red are the facets with the highest percentage.

Graph 1. Representation of the values obtained in each domain of the WHOQOL-brev.

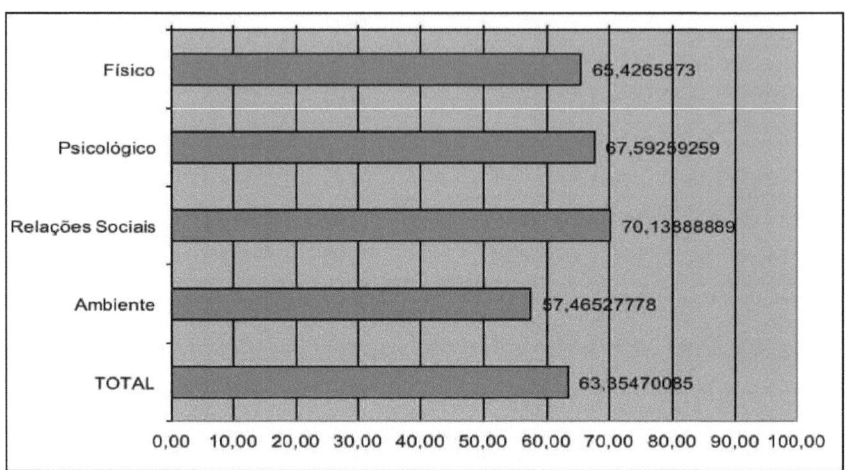

Source: Prepared by the researchers, database obtained from WHOQOL-brev (2016).

The Physical domain showed one of the worst values, but compared to the national average, it remained above 65%. And correlating the findings of each facet, the issue of pain and discomfort and the dependence on medication of these professionals is increasingly present. The lower values of the facets are within this domain, because in the day-to-day work of the nursing team it is common to find employees working in pain or using medication.

It can be inferred, based on Felli (2015), that nursing work is considered stressful due to work overload, with pressure on the time taken to perform tasks, causing an acceleration in the pace of work, exposure to risks and the development of occupational diseases. As a result, the activities performed result in high levels of fatigue that reduce work capacity.

The symptoms of fatigue are referred to as drowsiness, restlessness and lack of willingness to work, difficulty thinking, decreased attention, slowness, dulling of perceptions and decreased desire to work (SILVA et al., 2015). It is worth highlighting the phenomenon of presenteeism in everyday nursing work, as it differs from absenteeism, which is more easily measured by absences from work. Presenteeism refers to a work situation in which the worker remains present in the workplace, even though they are not achieving their ideal productivity, whether for personal, physical or mental reasons (FELLI, 2015).

Silva (2011) emphasizes that presenteeism means that sick people are working without complaining, without seeking treatment, while their medical conditions worsen and become more chronic, resulting in wear and tear that has a direct impact on the performance of their work activities.

From this perspective, knowing that night work is more harmful to workers' health, specifically that of nursing professionals, unfolds as the lack of adequate sleep and rest, having as a direct consequence the other facets being influenced, because the energy for the activities of daily life and work capacity are diminished and / or reduced.

According to a study by the Ministry of Labor, daytime sleep does not compensate in quantity and quality for the hours not slept at night, with a variety of consequences, such as greater predisposition to diseases linked to low immunity, changes in metabolic activity, obesity, headaches, among countless others (BRASIL, 2001).

In many workplaces, nursing professionals who work at night do not have adequate places to rest, and even though the country is continental in size, there is a huge lack of places for this purpose. It is important to mention the gains made by the profession with the approval of the Bill (PLS 597/2015), which provides for decent rest conditions for nursing professionals during working hours.

As a result, dependence on medication and/or treatment is a harsh reality: professionals who look after the lives of others are not concerned about their own health.

According to data from the WHO (2015), sick leave for workers has increased due to the effects of work overload, as have symptoms of stress, anxiety and depression. This has led to an increase in the use of medication and mood stabilizers. In addition to an increase in the number of absences due to mental and behavioral disorders, according to data from the Ministry of Labor and Social Security (FRAGA et al., 2016).

Graph 2. Representation of the values obtained in each facet of the WHOQOL-brev.

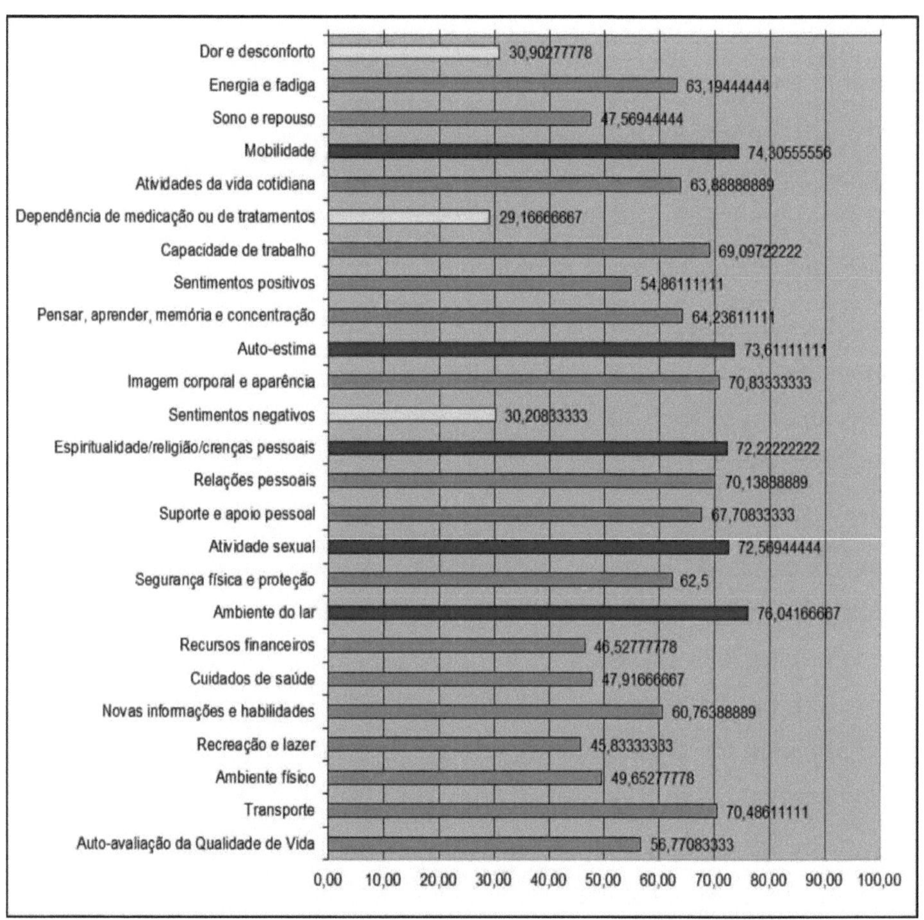

Source: Prepared by the researchers, database obtained from WHOQOL-brev (2016).

The Psychological domain scored the second highest among the others. In this domain, we can say that the group is average, with a good quality of life. The least representative facet was negative feelings.

There is a great difficulty in carrying out user care smoothly and with good results, either due to a lack of supplies and materials, or due to management and structural problems, which leads to feelings of concern and impotence on the part of nursing professionals (BRAGA et al., 2015).

At the same time, these feelings are influenced by other factors, as night work alters the rhythm of many organs, because the body's metabolic cycles, some hormones that stabilize mood, growth, such as cortisol, which should be secreted during sleep, stop being produced, altering and leaving an emotional instability causing reflections of mental exhaustion in the worker (JANSEN, 2007).

The number of hours worked in shifts is very controversial, as the human body can generally tolerate shifts of up to 12 hours, and it is very important to follow the recommendations in order to maintain physical integrity and safety at work. Considering that the best schedule will always be the one that is most consistent with the worker's daily routine, we are far from the reality of the nursing profession.

A study by Linda et al. (2014) reveals that over 90% of the most serious accidents in companies happen at night. In Brazil, accidents at work are still very common, and illness and working conditions are imposed by contracts and working hours. Brazilian nursing does not have a national salary floor, nor does it have a common working day, and it has sought to regulate the Law of 30 hours a week for all professionals.

Workers have been subjected to different workloads that generate processes of exhaustion or illness, compromising the health and lives of nursing staff, patients and the quality of care (FELLI, 2015).

The Social Relationships domain was the one that achieved the best value, reflecting directly on the general domain. This can be credited to the fact that the majority of the study population was married (58.3%), a fact identified in the results of the correlations between the variables.

The time structure of work is quite rigid: the longer the working day, the less time there is for family life and the greater the fatigue, the greater the strain on the quality of the worker's relationship with their family. There was a significant association between the long working hours of professionals and the lack of time for rest, leisure and socializing. And when the work is done at night, the need to sleep during the day and the fact that they are away from home at night disrupts relationships, causing conflicts (SILVA, 2011).

The long working hours, expressed by double employment or overtime, make sociability difficult, as the activity consumes a large portion of the time when they could be doing personal and domestic activities, for rest, leisure and family life. This absence increases levels of tension and anxiety, contributing to the prevalence of stress among nursing workers (FELLI, 2015).

On the other hand, Karino et al. (2015) cites that in the current context of nursing professionals, it can be seen that double work is a common practice, even though this choice can bring occupational risks, damage to their quality of life and to the care provided, as well as to self-care.

The Environment domain was characterized with the lowest average score, but its importance for understanding the reality experienced by the professionals in the nursing team is nonetheless evident.

Professionals in this team are exposed to countless harmful agents during their work, either because of the suffering they encounter on a daily basis, or because of the conflicts and problems within a multidisciplinary team with different characteristics and backgrounds. In addition, there are other cultural, structural, ergonomic and organizational interferences. Allied to physical, chemical, biological, mechanical, physiological and psychological risks and burdens.

Workers share the illness and death profiles of the general population, depending on their age, gender, social group or membership of specific risk groups. However, they can also fall ill or die from causes related to their work, as a result of their profession that they exercise or have exercised (BRASIL, 2001).

Nowadays, there is a lot of discussion about bullying and fear in the workplace. The 2013 Nursing Profile study showed that more than 70% of nursing professionals experience fear, anguish and situations of violence during their working day (COFEN/FIOCRUZ, 2013).

Felli (2012) points out that international statistics indicate that one in three nurses is likely to be subjected to physical or verbal abuse at work, compared to one in four police officers. In studies carried out in Brazil, prior to the one carried out by Fiocruz (2013), the rates were much higher: more than 80% of nursing professionals were affected by occupational violence.

Occupational diseases are illnesses directly related to the activity performed by the worker or due to the working conditions to which they are subjected (CORRÊA, 2015).

The majority of nursing work is done standing up, with a lot of moving around, in unsuitable positions and frequent handling of weights, substances and organic fluids, medicines and blood products, among countless others, which, together with other duties, cause fatigue, wear and tear and illness.

And this understanding is difficult to abstract because it is presented in a subjective way. And Horn and Contada (2011), when talking about this issue, state that subjectivity can be understood here as something internal and of an intimate nature, it happens from the group interaction to which the subject is subjected, in this environment the production of subjectivities is perceived. And when we talk about something subjective, we have to consider the risk factors in the employment contract: long working hours, shift work, low pay and the need for more than one employment relationship.

On the other hand, this demand is also pointed out by Linda et al. (2014), , who stated from a study in 9 European countries that most institutions and workplaces try to do more with less, causing serious deleterious consequences for nursing professionals. He also mentions that hospitals are constantly being targeted to reduce costs, causing concern about the quality of care and professional activities.

Corrêa (2015) states that one of the major ergonomic concerns in the workplace is body posture during work activities, which is related to the implications that a static or displaced position for several hours at a time can have. This is because inadequate conditions or postures can contribute to various types of damage, ranging from discomfort to pain and muscle problems.

But by trying to bring together the various themes that emerged from the domains and their facets, we can consider that listening, observing workers, taking a closer look at the events and meanings of conflicts in the workplace is a starting point for changing a reality.

Sato (2009), faced with this situation, suggested the process of "micro-negotiations" as a process of argumentation and counter-argumentation with the whole team, developing contexts that are present in daily life that can be changed and improved, and having, with the negotiations, subsidies to identify and change within the possibilities, thus minimizing the damage and conflicts in the work environment.

However, recognizing the role of work in determining and evolving the health-disease process of workers has ethical, technical and legal implications, which are reflected in the organization and provision of health actions for this segment of the population.

From this perspective, establishing the causal link between a given health event, be it injury or illness, and a given working condition is a basic condition for implementing health actions for workers in health services (BRASIL, 2001).

FINAL CONSIDERATIONS

The aim of this study was to analyze the impact of night work on the quality of life of male nursing professionals, using a questionnaire validated by the World Health Organization. Once the data was in hand, it had to be analyzed and grouped, thus achieving the proposed objective.

Through the research, it was possible to problematize and deconstruct some concepts of work relations, gender, quality of life and night work in the context of the nursing team. It also looked at the representations and discourses that deal with health care, especially the contours that exist within the nursing profession as part of gender relations.

With regard to representations, the professionalization and inclusion of men in the nursing team was a guiding factor, seeking to insert, demonstrate and correlate the importance of analyzing a significant and very present part of the daily life of many health teams in a hospital environment, by means of a gender and work shift.

With regard to the subjects' characteristics, there was a predominance of married couples, 42 (58.3%); 50 (69.4%) under a single legal employment contract, with an average age of 40 and 16 years' service. This scenario allowed for a better assessment of the domains and facets related to social relations.

It was very important to use the quality of life assessment tool, because measuring and treating its various facets and domains showed that the particularities related to their quality of life brought the relationship between the researcher and the participants closer, in order to understand a little of the reality they experienced and its reflexes and impacts on their state of health.

The research participants were very happy to take part in the study, feeling heard, represented and recognized when they answered the questionnaire, and the vast majority asked for *feedback* on the final study. This research, based on the data obtained, as well as the knowledge contextualized from the answers given by the participants, concludes that nursing work paradoxically contributes to a decrease in the quality of life of the professional, in terms of structures, conditions and risks at work.

This is because the work of nursing professionals is not always characterized by freedom, debate and creation, and because it is an activity governed by norms and takes place within rigidly defined parameters such as procedures, schedules and scales, the issue of the health of the worker and the team is left in the background.

Although the research was carried out in a single institution, we were able to verify its representativeness. This made it possible to generalize the results. This study had a limitation, since the quantitative approach did not allow for a more in-depth analysis of the issues, but it was possible to articulate and get to know better, through the questionnaire and its analysis, the trends and influences that impact on the quality of life of these professionals.

As we have seen in this paper, there are few studies that deal with gender within the nursing team and work shifts. As a result, in this study we have produced knowledge, within the possibilities and limitations, that will help us to find new ways of breaking with the arbitrary and cultural sexual division of labor that is present. In this way, we can reflect on the unequal social relations between subjects within the same activity.

We found evidence of an association between night work and quality of life in the population studied, and that some findings may also be related to those found in the facets, such as agreement between the different aspects present in the daily lives of these professionals.

It is suggested that further research be carried out with these professionals, using other methods or approaches, in order to identify the influences of shift work on their health. And by identifying the problems and conflicts, preventive plans can be drawn up, as well as measures to change the precarious reality in Brazilian health institutions.

And even though it is not possible to make a structural change in the nature of the nursing work object or to control its harmfulness, whether it is hazardousness, dangerousness or unhealthiness, it is possible to minimize its impacts with legal or managerial measures that distance the exposures or minimize the loads inherent in the night work performed by the nursing team.

Finally, we believe that this research can help inform future investigations, as nursing teams become aware of their importance and their work process, the risks, wear and tear, stress, work overload, as well as coping with health problems and harmful situations in the workplace, in order to reduce the consequences for workers.

In this way, the readings point to the need to provide better conditions and the necessary means so that they can change a common reality, aiming to glimpse and experience comfort, well-being, fulfillment and appreciation, belonging in the professional and personal spheres regardless of their gender or work shift, without this interfering with their quality of life and the quality of the care provided.

REFERENCES

ABREU, N.R. et al. Working night shifts: implications for workers' professional and personal quality of life. *Revista Gestao e tecnologia*. V.12, n.3. p.103-131, Sep./Dec. 2012. Available at: https://revistagt.fpl.edu.br/get/article/view/445. Accessed on: September 15, 2015.

AGUIAR, Z.N. Transformations in the process and organization of work and some implications for workers' health. In: RIBEIRO, M.C.S. (Org.). *Enfermagem e trabalho: fundamentos para a atenção à saù dos trabalhadores*. 2 ed. Sâo Paulo: Martinari, 2012.

ALBORNOZ, S. *O que é trabalho*. 6 ed. Sâo Paulo: Brasiliense, 2008. (Coleçâo primeiros passos).

ALVES, G. *Trabalho e subjetividade: o espirito do toyotismo na era do capitalismo manipulatório*. Sâo Paulo: Boitempo, 2011.

ALVES, G. *Trabalho e neodesenvolvimentismo: choque de capitalismo e nova degradaçao do trabalho no Brasil*. Bauru: Canal 6, 2014.

ALVES, G.; SANTOS, J.B.F. (Org.). *Research methods and techniques on the world of work*. Bauru: Canal 6, 2014.

ALVIM, M. B. Man's Relationship with Work in Contemporary Times; A Critical View Based on Gestalt Therapy. *Rev. Estud. Pesqui.*

Psychol., v.6, n. 2, p.122-130, 2006. Available at:< http://www.e-publicacoes.uerj.br/index.php/revispsi/article/viewFile/11031/8717 >, Accessed on: Dec. 10, 2015.

ANDRADE, M.L.A.G. Men's and women's health at work; a gender perspective. In: OLIVEIRA, E. M.(Org). *Work, health and gender in the age of globalization*. Goiânia: AB, 1997.

ANGELIM, R.C.M. Quality of life assessment using whoqol: bibliometric analysis of nursing production. *Revista Baiana de Enfermagem*, v.29, n.4, p.

400-410, Oct/Dec 2015. Available at:< http://search.proquest.com/openview/0964aa347e10a9e046bb19f38301c04f/1?pq-origsite=gscholar&cbl=2040112 >. Accessed on: Dec. 10, 2015.

ANTUNES, R. *Os sentidos do trabalho: ensaio sobre a afirmação e a negação do trabalhado.* 2 ed. Sâo Paulo: Boitempo, 2009.

ANTUNES, R. *Adeus ao trabalho? ensaio sobre a metamorfoses e a Centralidade do mundo do trabalho.* 16 ed. Sâo Paulo: Cortez, 2015.

ARENDT, H. *The human condition.* 12 ed. rev. Rio de Janeiro: Forense University, 2014.

BARATA, R. B. *Como e por que as desigualdades sociais fazem mal à saù?* Rio de Janeiro: Editora Fiocruz, 2009.

BARBOSA, E. S. et al. Men in nursing: the subjectivity of the nursing work process. *Rev. Lat. Enf.* Mar, p. 91-96, 2009. Available at:< http://www.revistas.usp.br/rlae/article/view/1557/0 >. Accessed on: 09 Dec 2015.

BARROS, A.L.B.L. et al. *Nursing process: guide to practice.* Sâo Paulo: COREN/SP, 2015.

BAUMAN, Z. *Liquid Modernity.* Trad. Plinio Dentzien. Rio de Janeiro: Zahar, 2001.

BAUMAN, Z. *Liquid Life.* Trad. Carlos Alberto Medeiros. 2 ed. Rio de Janeiro: Zahar, 2009.

BEUREN, I. (Org.) *Como elaborar trabalhos monogràficos em Contabilidade: teoria e pratica.* Sao Paulo: Atlas, 2 ed., 2004.

BOURDIEU, P. *A dominaçao masculina.* 9 ed. Rio de Janeiro: Bertrand Brasil, 2010.

BOUYER, G. C. Social and work-related suffering in the context of mental health and work. *Psicologia & Sociedade [online]*, v. 27, n.1, p. 116-119, 2015.

Available at:< http://www.scielo.br/pdf/psoc/v27n1/1807-0310-psoc- 27-01-00106.pdf >, Accessed on: 12 Dec. 2015.

BLAY, S.L. Design and methodology of quality of life research. In: DINIZ, D.P. et al. *Guia de qualidade de vida: saùde e trabalho*. Barueri, SP: Manole, 2013.

BRAGA, F. S.; OLSCHOWSKY, A. Pleasure and suffering in the work of mental health nurses in the context of psychiatric reform. *Revista de Enfermagem UFPE [online], v. 9, n. 3, p. 7086-7094, mar. 2015*. Available at: < http://www.lume.ufrgs.br/handle/10183/115332?locale=pt_BR >, Accessed on: Dec. 12, 2015.

BRAZIL. Ministry of Health. Pan American Health Organization in Brazil. *Work-related diseases: manual of procedures for health services.* Brasilia: Brazilian Ministry of Health, 2001. Available at: <

http://bvsms.saude.gov.br/bvs/publicacoes/doencas_relacionadas_trabalho1.pdf >, Accessed on: Sep. 10, 2015.

BRAZIL. Ministry of Health. Secretariat for Health Policies.

Department of Primary Care. *Workers' Health.* Brasilia: Ministry of Health, 2002.

BULHOES, I. *Riscos do trabalho* de *enfermagem*. 2 ed. Rio de Janeiro: Folha Carioca Editora, 1998.

BUSETTI, G. R. et al. *Saùde e qualidade de vida*. v.3. Sao Paulo; Peirópolis, 1998.

CARVALHO, G. M. *Enfermagem do Trabalho.* Sao Paulo: EPU, 2001.

CARVALHO. G.M. *Enfermagem do trabalho.* 2 ed. Rio de Janeiro: Guanabara Koogan, 2014.

CAVALCANTE, M. M.et al. Engagement, Well-Being at Work and Psychological Capital : a study with people management professionals. *Revista Pensamento & Realidade [online*], v. 29, n. 4, 2014. Available at:<

http://revistas.pucsp.br/index.php/pensamentorealidade/article/view/22391 >, Accessed on: September 10, 2015.

CHIAVENATO, I. *Recursos Humanos: o capital humano das organizaçôes*. 8 ed. Sao Paulo: Atlas, 2008.

CISNE, M. *Gènero, divisao sexual do trabalho e serviço social*. 1 ed. São Paulo: Ed. Outras Expressoes, 2012.

COFEN - Federal Nursing Council. *Survey of the profile of Brazilian nursing*. Available at:< http://www.cofen.gov.br/pesquisa- inedita-traca-perfil-da-enfermagem_31258.html >, Accessed on: 18 Dec. 2015.

COLUCCI, C. Violence in the workplace. *Folha de Sao Paulo*. Available at:< http://www1.folha.uol.com.br/cotidiano/2015/06/1639624-

70-of-nurses-in-the-country-don't-feel-safe-at-work.shtml >. Accessed on: 09 Dec. 2015.

CONNELL, R. *Gender: a global perspective*. Sâo Paulo: nVersos, 2015.

COREN/MG. *Regional Nursing Council of Minas Gerais. Legislation and Standards*. Belo Horizonte: COREN-MG, v.14, n.1,2015.

CORRÊA, V.M. *Ergonomics: fundamentals and applications*. Porto Alegre: Bookman, 2015.

COSTA, A.O. (Org). *Labor market and gender: internal comparisons*. Rio de Janeiro: Editora FGV, 2008.

COSTA, K.S. Presença masculina na escola de enfermagem da universidade de Sâo Paulo (1950-1990). *Rev. Cuidado, Fundam*. Oct/Dec, p. 203-207, 2010. Available at:< http://www.seer.unirio.br/index.php/cuidadofundamental/article/view/867 >.

Accessed on: Dec. 10, 2015.

CHERES, J.E.C. et al. *Night work: the inversion of the biological clock*. Available at: <

http://webcache.googleusercontent.com/search?q=cache:_yLPRQv9hu4J:fadipa.educacao.ws/ojs-2.3.3-3/index.php/cjuridicas/article/download/68/pdf+&cd=1&hl=en-BR&ct=clnk&gl=br >. Accessed on: January 12, 2016.

CZERESNIA, D. (Org.). *Health Promotion: concepts, reflections, trends.* 2 ed. rev. ampl. Rio de Janeiro: Editora Fiocruz, 2009.

DEJOURS, C. Towards a new concept of health. *Revista Brasileira de Saùde Ocupacional,* n. 54, vol.14. April-May-June,1986. Available at:< https://corepsp.files.wordpress.com/2010/05/apostila_formacao_saude_corep.pdf>. Accessed: Dec. 18, 2015.

DEJOURS, C. *Da psicopatologia à psicodinâmica do trabalho*. Editora Fiocruz, Brasilia, 2004.

DEJOURS, C. *The madness of work: a study of the psychopathology of work*. 6 ed. Sâo Paulo: Cortez, 2015.

DINIZ, D. P. et al. *Guide to quality of life: health and work*. Barueri, SP: Manole, 2013.

EBERHARDT, L. D. et al. Work relationship in the health sector: scenario of precariousness in the western macro-region of Paranà. *Revista Saùde Debate*, v.39, n.104, p.18-29, jan/mar 2015. Available at:< http://www.scielo.br/pdf/sdeb/v39n104/0103-1104-sdeb-39-104-00018.pdf >. Accessed on: December 10, 2015.

FANNGYI, G. U;. et al. Total and Cause-Specific Mortality of U.S. *Nurses Working Rotating Night Shifts. American Journal of Preventive Medicine* [online], v 48, issue 3, p. 241-252, 2015. . Available at:< http://www.ncbi.nlm.nih.gov/pubmed/25576495 >, Accessed on: Sep. 10, 2015.

FELLI, V.E.A. *Nursing working conditions and illness: reasons for reducing the working day to 30 hours*. Enfermagem em Foco, 2012. Available at:<

http://biblioteca.cofen.gov.br/wp- content/uploads/2016/02/Condicoes-de-trabalho-de-enfermagem-e- adoecimento.pdf >. Accessed on: 09 Dec. 2015.

FELLI, V. E. A. (Org.). *Health of the nursing worker*. Barueri, SP: Manole, 2015.

FERREIRA, M.C. *Qualidade de vida no trabalho: uma abordagem centrada no olhar dos trabalhadores*. 2 ed. Brasilia: Paralelo 15, 2012.

FILHO, G.I.R. *Ergonomia aplicada à odontologia: as doenças de caràter ocupacional em cirurgiao- dentista*. Curitiba: Editora Maio, 2004.

FILHO, N. A; ROUQUAYROL, M.Z. *Introduction to epidemiology*. 4 ed. revised and expanded. Rio de Janeiro: Guanabara koogan, 2014.

FILHO, A.J.A. et al. *Life history of Brazilian nurses: contribution to the development of nursing*. Brasilia: ABEn, 2016.

FIOCRUZ. Osvaldo Cruz Foundation. *Survey of the profile of Brazilian nursing.* Available at:< http://www.cofen.gov.br/pesquisa-inedita-traca- perfil-da-enfermagem_31258.html > . Accessed on: December 18, 2015.

FISCHER, F.M. et al. *Shift and night work in the 24-hour society*. Sào Paulo: Atheneu, 2003.

FLECK, M. P.A. et al. *Quality of life assessment: a guide for health professionals.* Porto Alegre: Artmed, 2008.

. *WHOQOL-Abbreviated.* Available at: < http://www.ufrgs.br/psiquiatria/psiq/whoqol84.html >. Accessed on: September 18, 2015.

FONTANA, R. T.; BRIGO, L. Studying and working: perceptions of nursing technicians about this choice. *Esc. Anna Nery* [online], v. 16, n. 1, p. 128133, 2012. Available at:< http://www.redalyc.org/articulo.oa?id=127721430017 >, Accessed on: September 9, 2015.

FONTELLES, M.J. *Bioestatistica aplicada à pesquisa experimental: volume 3.* Sao Paulo: Ed. Livraria da Fisica, 2012.

FOUCAULT, M. *History of sexuality: the will to know.* Sao Paulo: Paz & Terra, 2014.

FOUCAULT, M. *Vigiar e punir: nascimento da prisão.* 42 ed. Petrópolis, RJ: Vozes, 2014.

FRAGA, E. et al. *Worker absenteeism due to stress increases with the recession.* Available at;< http://www1.folha.uol.com.br/mercado/2016/07/1794750-afastamento-de-worker-leave-for-stress-increases-with-the-recession.shtml>. Accessed on: July 24, 2016.

FREIRE, P. *Pedagogia da autonomia: Saberes necessàrios a pràtica educativa.* 25 ed. Sao Paulo: Ed. Paz e Terra, 2002.

FREITAS, H., & MOSCAROLA, J. *From observation to decision: research methods and quantitative and qualitative data analysis.* RAE Eletrônica, 1(1), 1-29, 2002. Available at:< http://www.scielo.br/pdf/raeel/v1n1/v1n1a06 >, Accessed on: September 9, 2015.

FREUD, S. *O mal estar na civilizaçao [1930].* In: EDIÇÂO standard brasileira das obras psicológicas completas de Sigmund Freud. Rio de Janeiro: Editora Imago, 1976.

FUCHS, A.M.S. et al. *Guide to the standardization of technical and scientific publications.* Uberlândia: EDUFU, 2013.

GEOVANINI, T. et al. *History of nursing: versions and interpretations.* Rio de Janeiro: Revinter, 1995.

GERARDI, L.H.O. *Quantification in Geography.* Sâo Paulo: DIFEL, 1981.

HAAG, G.S. (Org.). *A enfermagem e a saùde dos trabalhadores.* 2 ed. Goiânia: AB, 2001.

HADDAD, N. *Metodologia e estudos em ciências da saù: como planejar, analisar e apresentar um trabalho cientifico.* Sâo Paulo: Roca, 2004.

HIRATA, H. *Nova divisao sexual do trabalho: um olhar voltado para a empresa e a sociedade*. Sâo Paulo: Boitempo Editorial, 2002.

HIRATA,H. KERGOAT, D. *New configurations of the sexual division of labor. Cadernos de pesquisa,* v. 37, n.132, p.595-609, Sep/Dec, 2007. Available at: < http://scielo.br/pdf/cp/v37n132/a0537132 >. Accessed on: 09 Dec. 2015.

HORN, C.H.; COTANDA, F.C.(Org). *Labor relations in the contemporary world: multidisciplinary essays*. Porto Alegre: Ed. UFRGS, 2011.

IBGE. Brazilian Institute of Geography and Statistics. *Brazil in numbers*. Available at: < http://www.ibge.gov.br/apps/populacao/projecao/ >. Accessed on December 12, 2015.

KARINO, M. E. et al. Workloads and fatigue of nursing workers in a teaching hospital. *Cienc Cuid Saude* [online], v. 14, n. 2, p. 1011-1018, 2015. Available at:< http://www.periodicos.uem.br/ojs/index.php/CiencCuidSaude/article/view/21603 >, Accessed on: September 9, 2015.

KIMURA, M. CARANDINA, M. Development and validation of a reduced version of the instrument for assessing the quality of life at work of nurses in hospitals. *Revista Escola de Enfermagem, USP*, 2009. Available at:< http://www.scielo.br/scielo.php?script=sci_arttext&pid=S0080-62342009000500008 >. Accessed on: Dec. 10, 2015.

JANSEN, J.M. (Org.). *Night medicine: from chronobiology to clinical practice*. Rio de Janeiro: Editora FIOCRUZ, 2007.

JOBS, E. *Where does innovation come from?* In: KAHNEY, L. A cabeça de Steve Jobs. 2ed, Rio de Janeiro: Agir, 2009.

LAKATOS, E.M.; MARCONI, M.A. *Fundamentos de Metodologia cientifica*. Sao Paulo: Atlas, 7 ed , 2010.

LINDA, H. A. et al. Nurse staffing and education and hospital mortality in nine European countries: a retrospective observational study. *The Lancet [online],*

v. 383, issue 993, 2014. Available at:< http://www.thelancet.com/journals/lancet/article/PIIS0140-6736(13)62631-8/abstract >, Accessed on: Oct. 9, 2015.

LOPES, M.J.M.et al. Persistent feminization in the professional qualification of Brazilian nursing. *Cadernos pagu*, jan/jun, p. 105-125, 2005.

Available at:< http://www.scielo.br/pdf/cpa/n24/n24a06.pdf >. Accessed on: 09 Dec. 2015.

LOBIONDO-WOOD, G.; et al. *Nursing research: methods, critical appraisal and utilization.* 4 ed. Rio de Janeiro: Guanabara Koogan. 2001.

LOBO, E.S. *The working class has two sexes: work, domination and resistance.* Sâo Paulo: Ed. Brasiliense, 1991.

LUONGO, J. (Org.). *Nursing at work*. Sâo Paulo: Rideel, 2012.

MACHADO, M.H. et al. General characteristics of nursing: the socio-demographic profile. *Revista Enfermagem* em foco, n.6, p.11-17, 2015. Available at: < http://revista.portalcofen.gov.br/index.php/enfermagem/article/view/686 >. Accessed on; 10 Dec. 2015.

MACHADO, M.H. et al. Nursing labor market: general aspects. *Revista Enfermagem em foco*, n.6, p.43-78, 2015. Available at:< http://biblioteca.cofen.gov.br/mercado-de-trabalho-da-enfermagem-aspectos-gerais/ >. Accessed on; 10 Dec. 2015.

MACHADO, M.H. et al. Nursing working conditions. *Revista Enfermagem em foco*, n.6, p.79-90, 2015. Available at:< http://biblioteca.cofen.gov.br/condicoes-de-trabalho-da-enfermagem/ >. Accessed on; Dec. 10, 2015.

MARTINO, M.M.F.; SILVA, C.A. Study of the chronotype of a group of shift workers. *Rev. bras. saùde ocup.* 2005, vol.30, n.111, pp. 1724. Available at:< http://periodicos.puc-campinas.edu.br/seer/index.php/cienciasmedicas/article/viewFile/1322/1296 >, Accessed on: September 10, 2015.

MARTINS, C.O. *PPST- Programa de promoçao da saù do trabalhador. 1* ed. Jundiai, SP: Ed. Fontoura, 2008.

MARTINS, C. C.F.; et al. Interpersonal relationship of the nursing team x stress: limitations for practice. *Cogitare Enfermagem*, v. 19, n. 2, 2014. Available at:< http://revistas.ufpr.br/cogitare/article/view/36985 >, Accessed on: September 9, 2015.

MARUANI, M.; HIRATA, H. (Org). *The new frontiers of inequality: men and women in the labor market*. Sao Paulo: Ed. Senac, 2003.

MARX, K. *Capital*. Rio de Janeiro: Civilizacao Brasileira, Book I, v. 2, 10th edition, 1985.

MELO, C. *Social division of labor and nursing*. Sao Paulo: Cortez, 1986.

MELO, L. P. (Org.). *Enfermagem, antropologia e saùde*. 1 ed. Barueri, SP: Manole, 2013.

MINAYO, M. C. S. *O desafio do conhecimento*. Sao Paulo: Editora Hucitec, 9ª. ed. revised and improved, 2006.

MINEO, J.R. et al. *Research in the biomedical field: from planning to publication.* Uberlândia: EDUFU, 2005.

MIRANDA, C.R. *Introduçao à saùde no trabalho*. Sao Paulo: Atheneu Publishing House, 1998.

NARDI, H.C. (Org). *Sexual diversity, gender relations and public policies.* Porto Alegre: Sulina, 2013.

NEFFA, J. C. Human work and its centrality. *Revista Ciências do Trabalho [online],* n. 4, 2015. Available at:< http://rct.dieese.org.br/rct/index.php/rct/article/view/85 >, Accessed on: 9 Oct. 2015.

NERI, A.L. (Org.). *Qualidade de vida e idade madura. 7 ed. Campinas/SP: Papirus, 2007.*

NOBREGA, J. S. The issue of workers' health in self-managed enterprises. *Caderno de Psicologia Social do Trabalho*, v.17, n.1, p.129142, 2014. Available at: <

http://pepsic.bvsalud.org/pdf/cpst/v17n1/a10v17n1.pdf >. Accessed on: December 10, 2015.

NOGUEIRA, C.M. *O trabalho duplicado: a divisa sexual no trabalho e na reproduçâo: um estudo das trabalhadoras do telemarketing. 2* ed. Sao Paulo: Expressao Popular, 2011.

NOLASCO, S. *De Tarzan a Homer Simpson: banalizaçao e violência masculina em sociedades contemporâneas ocidentais*. Rio de Janeiro: Rocco, 2001.

NOVARETTI, A.C.Z. et al. Nursing work overload and adverse events and incidents in ICU patients. *Rev. Bras. Enferm.* Sep/Oct, 2014. Available at: < http://www.scielo.br/scielo.php?script=sci_arttext&pid=S0034-71672014000500692 >. Accessed on; 10 Dec. 2015.

OGUISSO, T. *O exercicio da enfermagem: uma abordagem ético-legal.* 2 ed. atual. e ampl. Rio de Janeiro: Guanabara Koogan, 2007.

OGUISSO, T. (Org.). *Historical and legal trajectory of nursing.* Sao Paulo: Manole, 2007.

OLIVEIRA, E.M.(Org). *Work, health and gender in the age of globalization.* Goiânia: AB, 1997.

OLIVEIRA, M. L.; PAULA, T. R.; FREITAS, J B. Historical evolution of nursing care. *Conscientia e Saùde*, v. 6, n. 1, p.:127-36, 2007. Available at:< http://www.redalyc.org/articulo.oa?id=92960115 >, Accessed on: October 9, 2015.

OLIVEIRA, R.G. (Org.). *BlackBook- Enfermagem*. Belo Horizonte: BlackBook Editora, 2016.

WHO. *World Health Organization*. Available at:< http://www.who.int/eportuguese/countries/bra/pt/ >. Accessed on: 12 Dec. 2015.

PAFARO, R. C.; MARTINO, M. M. F.. Study of the stress of nurses working double shifts in a pediatric oncology hospital in Campinas. *Rev esc enferm USP*, v. 38, n. 2, p. 152-60, 2004. Available at: < http://www.revistas.usp.br/reeusp/article/viewFile/41391/44970 >, Accessed on: Oct. 9, 2015.

PEDROSO, B. PILATTI, L.A. *Avaliação de indicadores da área da saúde: a qualidade de vida e suas variantes*. FAFIT/FACIC, Itararé-SP, 2010.

Available at: <http://www.fafit.com.br/revista/index.php/fafit/article/view/2>. Accessed on: 10 Dec. 2015.

PEREIRA, A.V. Relaçôes de gènero no trabalho: reflexoes a partir de imagens construidas de enfermeiros e enfermeiras. *Cad. Esp. Fem.* Uberlândia/MG, v.24, n.1,p. 49-77, jan/jun. 2011. Available at:< http://www.seer.ufu.br/index.php/neguem/article/view/14218 >, Accessed on: 10 Dec. 2015.

PEREIRA, P.F. *Homens na enfermagem: atravessamentos de gênero da escolha, formação e exercício profissional. (Dissertaçao)*. Porto Alegre, 2008. Available at:< http://www.lume.ufrgs.br/bitstream/handle/10183/13069/000639229.pdf? >, accessed on: October 9, 2015.

PIGNATI, W.A.; et al. Workers' Health. In: ROUQUAYROL, M.Z.; GURGEL, M. *Epidemiologia e saùde*. 7 ed. Rio de Janeiro; Medbook, 2013.

PINHEIRO,T.M.M.; et al. Workers' Health. In: CAMPOS, G.W.S. (Org). *Tratado de saùde coletiva*. 2 ed. rev. aum. Sao Paulo: Hucitec, 2012.

POLIT, D.F. *Fundamentals of nursing research: method, evaluation and utilization.* 5 ed. Porto Alegre: Artmed, 2004.

REGIS FILHO, G. I. *Ergonomics applied to dentistry: occupational diseases in dental surgeons*. Curitiba: Editora Maio, 2004.

REY, F.G. *Subjectivity and health; overcoming the clinic of pathology*. Sao Paulo: Cortez, 2011.

ROCHA, G.C. *Trabalho, saùde e ergonomia: relação entre aspectos legais e médicos.* 6 ed. Curitiba: Juruà, 2012.

ROCHA, M.I.B. (Org). *Work and gender: changes, continuities and challenges.* Sao Paulo: Ed.34, 2000.

RODRIGUES, A. *Psicologia Social*. Petrópolis, RJ: Vozes, 27 ed. rev. e ampl.. 2009.

RODRIGUES, M. R.; BRETAS, A. C. P. *Ageing at work from the perspective of nursing workers*. Trab. educ. saùde

[online], v. 13, n. 2, p. 343-360, 2015. Available at: < http://www.scielo.br/scielo.php?script=sci_arttext&pid=S1981-77462015000200343 >Accessed on: September 10, 2015.

ROHM, R. H. D.; LOPES, N. F. R . The new meaning of work for the postmodern subject: a critical approach. *Cad. EBAPE.br[online],* v. 13, n. 2, art. 6, Rio de Janeiro, Apr./Jun. 2015. . Available at:< http://www.scielo.br/pdf/cebape/v13n2/1679-3951-cebape-13-02-00332.pdf >, Accessed on: October 10, 2015.

ROLIM, K. I.; WENDLING, M. I. The story of the two of us: reflections on the formation and dissolution of conjugality. *Psychol. clin. [online*], v. 25, n. 2, p. 165-180, 2013. Available at:< http://www.scielo.br/scielo.php?script=sci_arttext&pid=S0103-56652013000200010 >, Accessed on: October 10, 2015.

ROTENBERG, L. et al. Gender and night work: Sleep, daily life and experiences of those who exchange night for day. *Cad. Saùde Pùblica*, Rio de Janeiro, 17, 639-649, mai-jun, 2001. Available at:< http://www.scielo.br/scielo.php?pid=S0102-311X2001000300018&script=sci_abstract&tlng=en >. Accessed on: December 10, 2015.

ROUQUAYROL, M. Z.; SILVA, M. G. C. *Epidemiologia & saùde*. 6 ed. Rio de Janeiro: MedBook, 2003.

ROUQUAYROL, M. Z.; SILVA, M. G. C. *Epidemiologia & saùde*. 7 ed. Rio de Janeiro: MedBook, 2013.

SANTANNA, A. S. *Qualidade de vida no trabalho: fundamentos e abordagens.* Rio de Janeiro: Elsevier, 2011.

SANTOS, M. *Por uma outra Globalizaçao do pensamento ùnico à consciência universal.* Editora Record: Rio de Janeiro, 9 ed. 2002.

SATO, L. Prevention of occupational health problems: redesigning work through daily negotiations. *Cad. Saùde Pùblica*. Rio de Janeiro, 2002. Available at:< http://www.scielo.br/pdf/csp/v18n5/10988.pdf >, Accessed on: September 10, 2015.

SATO, L. Work: suffering: building up? Resist? *Psicologia em Revista*, Belo Horizonte, v. 15, n.3, p.189-199, 2009. Available at: <

http://pepsic.bvsalud.org/pdf/per/v15n3/v15n3a12.pdf>. Accessed on: 10 Dec. 2015.

SEIDL, E. M. Quality of life and health: conceptual aspects and methodological . *Cad. Saùde Pùblica*. 2004, vol.20, n.2, pp. 580-588. . Available at:< http://www.scielo.br/pdf/csp/v20n2/27.pdf >, Accessed on: October 9, 2015.

SEVERINO, A. J. *Metodologia do trabalho cientifico*. 23 ed. rev. e atual. Sâo Paulo: Cortez, 2007.

SILVA, A.A. ROTENBERG, L. FISCHER, F.M. Working hours in nursing: between individual needs and working conditions. *Rev. Saùde Pùblica,* v.45, 2011. Available at:< http://www.scielo.br/scielo.php?script=sci_arttext&pid=S0034-89102011000600014 >. Accessed on: December 10, 2015.

SILVA, E. S. *Trabalho e desgaste emocional: o direito de ser dono de si mesmo.* Cortez, Sâo Paulo, 2011.

SILVA, M. A. *Discussing gender through work.* Available at:< http://www.portalanpedsul.com.br/admin/uploads/2012/Genero,_Sexualidade_e_Educacao/Trabalho/12_37_49_439-7454-1-PB.pdf >. Accessed on: December 10, 2015.

SILVA, R.M. et al. Night work and the repercussions on nurses' health. *Esc. Anna Nery,* 2011 Apr-Jun:15(270-279). Available at: <http://www.scielo.br/pdf/ean/v10n3/v10n3a06>. Accessed on: December 10, 2015.

SILVA, R.M. Morning, afternoon or indifferent? Knowledge production on chronotype in nursing. *Rev. Enfermagem UFSM,* 2014 Oct/Dec. Available at:< http://periodicos.ufsm.br/reufsm/article/view/12888 >.

Accessed on:Dec. 10, 2015.

SOUZA, L.L. et al. Representations of gender in nursing practice from the perspective of students. *Rev. Ciência & Cogniçao*, 2014; v.19, p.218-232. Available at: <

http://www.cienciasecognicao.org/revista/index.php/cec/article/viewFile/908/pdf_13 >. Accessed on: 10 Dec. 2015.

TURKIEWICZ, M. *History of nursing*. Paranà: Etecla, 1995.

TORRES, J.S.P. et al. *The male quantitative profile of nursing in Rondônia, Brazil.* Available at:< http://www.revistaintertexto.com.br/adm/arquivos/Artigo-

O%20PERFIL%20QUANTITATIVO%20MASCULINO%20DA%20ENFERMAGEM%20EM%20RONDÔNIA,%20BRASIL-Edicao-24-3132014-H141949-OPERFILQUANTITATIVOMASCULINODAENFERMAGEMEMRONDÔNIA,BRASIL.pdf >. Accessed on: December 10, 2015.

VIEIRA, S. *Metodologia cientifica para a àrea da saùde. 2* ed. Rio de Janeiro: Elsevier, 2015.

VITORINO, D.F.P. et al. Perception of male nursing professionals by residents of a city in Minas Gerais. *Rev. Min. Enferm.* v.16, p. 528-538, Oct/Dec, 2012. Available at:< http://www.reme.org.br/artigo/detalhes/558 >. Accessed on: December 10, 2015.

ZAR, J. H. Biostatistical analysis. 4 ed. Englewood Cliffs: Prentice Hall, 1999.

APPENDICES

APPENDIX A - FREE AND INFORMED CONSENT FORM FOR PARTICIPATION IN THE STUDY

You are being invited to take part in the research entitled "Impact of night work on the quality of life of male nursing professionals", under the responsibility of researchers Rafael Lemes de Aquino and Ailton de Souza Aragâo. In this research we are seeking to understand and evaluate the impact on the quality of life of male night nursing workers. The Informed Consent Form will be obtained by the researcher, Rafael Lemes de Aquino, and will be carried out in the participant's own work sector, within the Hospital de Clinicas of the Federal University of Uberlândia. You will be asked to fill in a questionnaire containing 26 questions, read each question, see what you think and circle the number that seems to be the best answer, the numbers are: 1 (very bad), (2) bad, (3) neither bad nor good, (4) good, (5) very good. You only have to choose the option that best suits you. At no time will you be identified. The results of the survey will be published and your identity will be preserved. You will not incur any financial costs for taking part in the study. The risks associated with this study consist of the possible identification of the research subjects, however, these risks will be mitigated because at no time will you be identified, noting also that the collection instrument only contains the following fields: age, marital status, position, employment relationship and length of service. As far as direct physical or moral risks are concerned, there are no risks to them, nor to the professionals involved, nor to the institution where the study will be carried out. Confidentiality will be guaranteed with regard to personal identification and the patient's willingness to take part in the study or not. The executing team is committed to absolute confidentiality regarding the identity of the research subject and their personal information. The results of the research will be of direct benefit to the scientific community and the care team, as obtaining this data will make it possible to characterize and manage health information, enabling the implementation of health and safety programs at work, as well as helping in the organization and structuring of health services. The researchers will treat the identity of the participants with professional standards and in accordance with CNS Resolution 466/12. You are free to stop taking part in the research at any time without any prejudice or coercion. You will keep an original copy of this Informed Consent Form. If you have any questions about the research, you can contact: Rafael Lemes de Aquino - (34) 3218-2071 - Av. Para, 1720 - Campus Umuarama - Uberlândia/MG and/or Ailton de Souza Aragâo - (34) 33185500, Av. Getûlio Guarità, 159. Sala 324, Universidade Federal do Triângulo Mineiro. You can also contact the Ethics Committee for Research with Human Beings - Federal University of Uberlândia: Av. Joâo Naves de Âvila, no 2121, bloco A, sala 224, Campus Santa Mônica - Uberlândia -MG, CEP: 38408-100; phone: 34-32394131.

RAFAEL LEMES DE AQUINO AILTON DE SOUZA ARAGÂO

Researchers' signatures

I agree to take part in the above-mentioned project voluntarily, after having been duly informed.

Research participant

APPENDIX B

data collection form - questionnaire

ADDRESS; MARITAL STATUS:POSITION:V | NCULO:TIME OF SERVICE:

So, go through each question, see what you come up with and circulate .

1 (multo ru m), (2) bad, (3) neither bad nor good. (4) good, (5) very good

1. Coma vacs avallarla sua quai Idade de vida? **113 4 S**

{1 i⁽⁰⁾r|uito InaatisreiEck₁ (ZJ ir|≡√Hii∊lto, (3}πerr| EJHisleito nem ΛsabsΓ⅛1c|. (41 BatiBfeita₁ (5) r∏uita Saliefeite

2. QUBO ≡ati ≡feitc | (a] VOOB is with your health? **1134 5**

The following questions are about how much vacancy there is in the last few weeks.

(2) mu ita pauco₁ 3) mais ou meπc | Ξ, (4) bastante, (5) ejdʳemameπ1e

3. In what πieditEa do you think your (physical) pain prevents you from doing what you need to do?

4. How much medical treatment do you need to go about your daily life? **12 345**

5. How much do you enjoy life? **1234 5**

Б. To what extent do you think the sub-life reads SBntido? **1234 5**

7. How well can you concentrate? **1234 5**

8. HOW safe DO you feel in your daily life? **1234 5**

9. How bad is your physical environment (climate, noise, pollution, allergens)? **12 345**

| The following questions will allow YOU to know how completely YOU are able or willing to work.

of making certain Arises ∏eztas Liltimas dja≡ zema∏ as.

{1) naca. (2) fine peйсе, {3) average, (4} mu ita, (5} cam Cletamenle

10. Do you have enough energy for your day-to-day life? **12 3 4 5**

11. Can you accept Bua's physical appearance? **1234 5**

12. Voca lem di nt⅝eiro SirficiE nt E para ≡ali≡fazer suas nacass Idades? **12 3 4 5**

13. How available is the information you need in your daily life? **12 3 4 5**

14. To what extent do you have leisure activity opportunities? **1234 5**

The following questions ask how well or satisfactorily you feel about

various aspects of his life in the LH but d jas вeтanaв.

{1) a lot of ru im. (2) ru im, (3) neither ru Im nor good. (4) bcm m ui1□, (5) barn

15. How well can you move? **12 3 4 5**

{1) mu to irsati≡fBrlα (2) in Batisfeiici, (3) nem sai'Ffeitc пвт Insatisfeilo₁ 4) satisfeitc | , (5) mu to sa1isfeitα

16. How satisfied are you with your sleep? **12 3 4 5**

17. How satisfied□{a} you are сот в your ability to carry out the activities of the **12 3 4 5**

your day-to-day life?

18. How satisfied | a) are you with your ability for work? **12 3 4 5**

19. How satisfied are you? **12 3 4 5**

29. How satisfied are you with your relationships with people (friends, relatives, colleagues)?

30. How satisfied are you with your sex life? **1234 5**

31. How satisfied are you with the cake you receive from your friends? **12 345**

32. How satisfied are you with the conditions in the locat where you live? **1234 5**

33. How satisfied are you with your access to healthcare? **12 3 4 5**

34. How satisfied are you your means of transportation? 12345 **12345**

The following questions refer to how often you felt ou experimeriou osrias

QpigBS nas. The last two versions,.

{1) ∏u∏ca, (2) a | gumag times. (3) f.'eq Lientemerte, (4) muilo freqùenleme nte. (5} always

35. How often do you have negative feelings such as bad moods? **12 3 4 5**

dieses pero, a∏siedade, tfepressâ?

Did anyone help you fill in this questionnaire?

How long did it take you to complete this questionnaire?

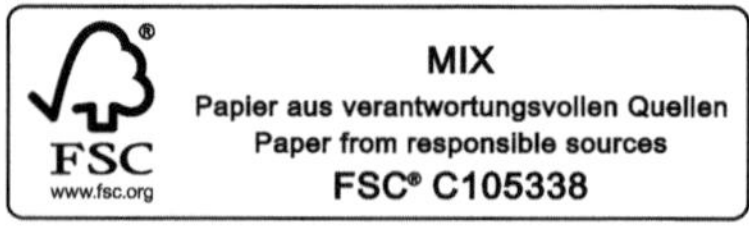

Printed by Books on Demand GmbH, Norderstedt / Germany